Herbal Intellig

"*Herbal Intelligence* is a brilliant work with surprising insights. It provides deep historical context for people's herbalism while challenging us to take personal responsibility. As we witness the collapse of various systems—ecosystems, societal structures, health care—it urges us to 'build a resilient medicine chest.' David has given us a practical guide on how local herbs, herbalism, and community herbalists can play a meaningful role in survival and resilience in these increasingly uncertain times."

J. A. BRINCKMANN, PRESIDENT OF THE BOARD OF TRUSTEES AT THE AMERICAN BOTANICAL COUNCIL AND VICE CHAIR OF THE BOTANICAL DIETARY SUPPLEMENTS AND HERBAL MEDICINES EXPERT COMMITTEE AT THE UNITED STATES PHARMACOPOEIA

"This book calls for a revolution, a green revolution. It delves into history, plant chemistry, synergy, new and old ideas, philosophy, ecology, and politics. It lays out the foundation for the use of herbs for personal, community, and global health, while breaking the links between the commodification and industrialization of plant medicine and our relationship with plants as our oldest allies in healing."

DAVID WINSTON, RH(AHG), AUTHOR OF *ADAPTOGENS*

"This book is on the cutting edge of herbalist knowledge. It explores the subject from its Paleolithic beginnings all the way to the research results of modern analytic science, while at the same time not forgetting holistic ecological aspects and the sacredness of life."

WOLF D. STORL, PHD, AUTHOR OF *THE HEART AND ITS HEALING PLANTS* AND *WITCHCRAFT MEDICINE*

"It's a joy to be ensnared in David Hoffmann's web. Want to reweave the healing cloak of the ancients? Read this book from one of the century's brightest minds and greenest hearts. As a green witch, I've long admired his green man persona. As a trained scientist, I've long applauded his clear thinking and clear speech. Read any part of *Herbal Intelligence*, and you'll applaud and admire him too."

SUSUN WEED, AUTHOR OF THE WISE WOMAN HERBAL SERIES

"This book is infused with joy, reverence, and hope. Underpinning it all is our everlasting relationship with plants, grounded in simple daily rhythms of the herbal practice. If you haven't explored herbalism, David tells why you need to and lays out a variety of entry paths: from the systems science that is helping us better understand the wild complexity of plant chemistry in medicine, to an ecologically grounded philosophy that suggests these plants can connect us to planetary intelligence in a meaningful way, to a basic tool kit of herbal remedies you can make and use yourself. David shows how herbal intelligence can help us today and serve as a life raft for the future."

GUIDO MASÉ, CLINICAL HERBALIST, HERBAL EDUCATOR,
AND AUTHOR OF *THE WILD MEDICINE SOLUTION*

"David Hoffmann has been present at every seminal juncture for herbalists, and with *Herbal Intelligence*, he once again delivers vital teachings with brilliance and bravery. From seeding true holism into our herbal work with his early books to delving deeper into the magnificence of science with *Medical Herbalism*, Hoffmann now guides our community and the world with grace, integrity, and uncanny tenderness through the storms and stunning possibilities of these challenging times."

KAT MAIER, FOUNDER AND DIRECTOR OF
SACRED PLANT TRADITIONS AND AUTHOR OF *ENERGETIC HERBALISM*

"David Hoffmann has once again written a masterful tome for herbalists everywhere! This philosophical and practical look into botanical medicine spans its historical roots into the 21st century and beyond. From our human relationship with the planet and its medicine all the way to an herbal primer, this is yet another indispensable classic for every herbalist's bookshelf."

SAM COFFMAN, RH, FOUNDER AND DIRECTOR OF THE
HERBAL MEDICS ACADEMY AND AUTHOR OF *HERBAL MEDIC*

"Hoffmann shows that the use of herbal remedies, which has taken place throughout history and everywhere on earth, is not only still fully valid but also the most beneficial way to cure illnesses."

CHRISTOPHER VASEY, ND, AUTHOR OF *THE NATUROPATHIC WAY* AND
THE ACID-ALKALINE DIET FOR OPTIMUM HEALTH

Herbal Intelligence

Plant Teachers and the
Return of Viriditas

David Hoffmann, FNIMH, RH

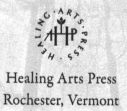

Healing Arts Press

Rochester, Vermont

Healing Arts Press
One Park Street
Rochester, Vermont 05767
www.HealingArtsPress.com

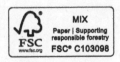

Healing Arts Press is a division of Inner Traditions International

Note to the reader: *This book is intended as an informational guide. The remedies,
approaches, and techniques described herein are meant to supplement, and not to be a
substitute for, professional medical care or treatment. They should not be used to treat a
serious ailment without prior consultation with a qualified health care professional.*

Cataloging-in-Publication Data for this title is available from the Library of Congress

ISBN 978-1-62055-614-6 (print)
ISBN 978-1-62055-615-3 (ebook)

Printed and bound in the United States by Lake Book Manufacturing, LLC

10 9 8 7 6 5 4 3 2 1

Text design and layout by Virginia Scott Bowman
This book was typeset in Garamond Premier Pro, Frutiger, and Gill Sans, with Span
and Neuzeit Grotesk used as display typefaces

To send correspondence to the author of this book, mail a first-class letter to the
author c/o Inner Traditions • Bear & Company, One Park Street, Rochester, VT
05767, and we will forward the communication.

Scan the QR code and save 25% at InnerTraditions.com.
Browse over 2,000 titles on spirituality, the occult, ancient
mysteries, new science, holistic health, and natural medicine.

Contents

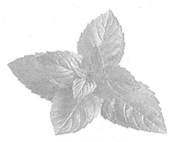

PREFACE

Radicle and Radical: My Path to Herbalism

These are special times—words fail trying to express the wonder and the horror of it all. In the face of ongoing global trauma, signs of transformation are manifesting; people are bringing the change. One of the causes for hope is the reappearance of herbalism—a reemergence that is not directed by the elites of science and medicine, not promoted as mass-media headline "'breakthroughs," but arising from a flowering in the cracks of our culture.

The path leading to the worldview that underpins this book has been long and convoluted. When I first started planning this book, I meant to use it to lay out my personal vision of how herbalism might contribute to the twenty-first century. Since that time, my views on herbalism have not changed, but the realities of the twenty-first century have blown away my complacency. Inculcated by "new age" wishful thinking combined with the zeal of the privileged would-be intellectual, I had envisioned the twenty-first century as a time of cultural renewal and the dawn of earth-centered medicine, politics, and economics. As it turns out, that vision was a fever dream of twentieth-century idealism. An honest assessment of what is hitting the fan leads to very different conclusions.

While the elite and those in power appear to be committed to the destruction of the planet, most people don't seem to care, having allowed themselves to be distracted by the media spectacle. Things are getting rapidly worse. I see little to have hope in, especially as it is often hope that things will get better that keeps us chained to the system that is causing the destruction. Hope of this kind is a deviously Machiavellian way of keeping us in line.

Today, the world's rulers—political, economic, or business—have no rational analysis of or explanation for the future. A small group of people now has more concentrated power over the human future than ever before in history, and they appear to have no vision, no strategy, no plan (or none they are willing to acknowledge). Whatever hope I had for the mainstream has been ripped away by the rictus grin of capitalism and the greed it nurtures. There are many facts to review and issues to consider, each with appropriate insights and conclusions. However, wherever we look, it is ever clearer that a breakdown is coming.

Given the current state of the world, the intent of the book has morphed into an exploration of how herbalism will help us cope with a dark and uncertain future.

My path to herbalism was incubated in England in the 1950s, during a very "post" part of the country's history. England was post war, post empire, post Holocaust, but a culture in shock, grief, and loss. The Final Solution of the Nazis had obliterated all of my father's family, like so many others, in the death camps and slave factories. He survived because he had been interned in a French concentration camp. Active in the antifascist ferment of Europe in the 1930s, he had joined the Czechoslovakian contingent of the volunteer International Brigades fighting Franco's fascists during the Spanish Civil War. Following Franco's victory, the International Brigades escaped over the Pyrenees into France. All these leftists, having come from a multitude of countries, were rounded up into concentration camps and not released until the outbreak of World War II.

I had little to no experience of nature in my childhood. A five-hundred-pound World War II German bomb created the "garden" I played in. I suppose my first intimation of *viriditas*, the divine, greening force of nature, came while I was hanging out with the fireweed (*Epilobium angustifolium*) in that bomb site. Looking back, I can see that it was a very magical place!

My first upwelling of resistance, characterized by incoherent adolescence, occurred during the Cuban missile crisis in 1962. As an eleven-year-old, I found myself in shock—the adults had totally messed up the world! My "elders and betters" were going to destroy everything. That feeling of disbelief and betrayal led me to sign the Peace Pledge, created after World War II by the Peace Pledge Union, a pacifist organization based in the United Kingdom. The pledge became an affirmation and stance in life that is central to all that I am even today. In its original phrasing, the pledge stated: "War is a crime against humanity. I renounce war and am therefore determined not to support any kind of war. I am also determined to work for the removal of all causes of war and campaign to promote peaceful and nonviolent solutions to conflict."

The young had no hope for a future unless we created it ourselves. I discovered the resistance, the cultural fringe, the oppressed I shared the planet with: my brothers around the world whom the elite would turn into cannon fodder, my sisters turned into brood hens for the machine, the workers in the "dark satanic mills" William Blake spoke of, people in the fields growing the crops that ensured affluence for their masters.

This dawning radicalization was saved from turning me into another casualty of the failed revolution by what turned into flower power—that is, revolution as celebration. My anarcho-syndicalism flowered into hippie craziness in the rich soil of the Summer of Love. The 14 Hour Technicolor Dream was on my birthday: April 29, 1967. This wild rock concert in London, a fund-raiser for the underground paper *International Times*, was probably as close as Britain came to matching the intensity and creativity of Ken Kesey's LSD-fueled Acid Tests in San Francisco.

I had been introduced to the tumult of rock and roll in the 1960s through my father, who was a photographer in the music industry of "swinging London." I had gone on tour with the Beatles in 1964 and had met the Rolling Stones, the Animals, and many others. By 1967 London was a cornucopia of raucous, transcendent, transformative music, a perfect accompaniment to the California sunshine that was then dawning. Music had become an international vehicle for change, a shared language of joyous transformation and revolution. By the end of the 1960s, I was in awe of life and Earth. The wonder of it all revealed by science was the same as the wonder of it all revealed by psychedelics. What a time to be alive!

Like so many others, I went on a personal journey to the East, following what became known as the hippie trail to Kathmandu. A story for another time. However, this transformative journey was also my first personal confrontation with fascism and the spirit of oppression. On the way out of Europe I stopped in Greece, at the time under the regime of a military junta known as "the Colonels." On the surface they were bumbling, incompetent, would-be strongmen, saving Greece from communism and the people. Living under their rule proved that the jackboot hurts no matter how clumsily it is worn.

When the movie *Woodstock* premiered in Athens, it triggered what the Greek media described as "confusion and public disorder," which was suppressed by the usual "police riots." I found myself involved in such things in Thessaloniki, in northern Greece. We happened to be there when the movie premiered in 1970 and so we went. The cinema was filled with hippies—it felt just like home—and the streets were patrolled by the police and army. When Sly and the Family Stone came on playing "Dance to the Music," the audience became ecstatic. In the film, Sly engaged the crowd in a call-and-response chant of "Higher!" and we all joined in as the music segued into "I Want to Take You Higher."

What we weren't expecting was the rest of the audience taking it into the street. The celebration turned into a street party, but the street belonged to the men with guns. It became a bloody melee. The eruption of joy threatened those in power—and they made us pay with our blood. Of course, I just continued on my way east (once the authorities allowed me to), but the rest of the audience couldn't.

The next stop, in Turkey, was even worse. The country was experiencing major internal conflict between the right and left, leading the police to patrol in groups of three for their own safety. It seemed that the only thing the various warring factions could agree on was that hippies were fair game. This was justified because our long hair was seen as an insult to women.

My next police riot was also in 1970 in Greece. The fascist Colonels had banned outdoor gatherings and restricted access to rock music, but in an attempt to attract tourists back to the country, they held music events with the classic-sounding name "Song Olympiads." Although they were clearly state propaganda and not rock festivals, the events usually had a Western rock component. In 1970 I attended one of these Song Olympiads, as a photographer helping my father. This meant I had free access backstage. It was held in the Panathenaic Stadium, a classical cultural monument. The modern Olympic Games were revived here in 1896, and the stadium is still the place from where the Olympic flame is handed over to the country hosting the games.

What had been a relatively boring event suddenly changed when a band from Scotland, called Marmalade, performed. Back home in the U.K. they were a middle-of-the-road pop band, but that night they channeled the revolution and celebration. The white marble stands suddenly lit up with dancing and joy. I was among the military elite—medals and machine guns—and I realized they were freaking out and directing the forcible suppression of people in the stadium and outside. It was another response of violence to quell celebration. The situation got bad, but I was saved by a police bus taking "guests" back to their hotels!

In 1970 I began studying biological sciences at the University of Sussex in Brighton. My life at university was characterized by a degree of undergraduate radicalism that, looking back, is embarrassing to behold! However, my classmates and I achieved a number of interesting things. The whole campus was forced into a reevaluation of course structures, grading systems, and educational goals. (Of course, a couple of years later much of it was quietly forgotten as we graduated and moved on to cause trouble elsewhere.)

An example of radical zeal confronting science education was my involvement in frog liberation! One of my first courses was Biochemistry 101, in which students had to kill and dissect frogs to extract the diaphragm in order to gain access to mitochondria-rich cells and thus explore the biochemistry of ATP (adenosine triphosphate). Educationally, the protocol offered many meaningful teaching moments. However, for most of the students, this was their first dissection. When presented with a bucket of frogs from which they each had to choose which one to kill, the whole class indignantly refused. As it turns out, the same biochemistry could be done with potatoes. The frogs were used simply to desensitize future biologists. To learn about life, we had to kill it!

In 1973 a mass boycott prevented the U.S. military apologist Samuel Huntington from lecturing on campus. His views on the Vietnam War, and especially his work as a strategic advisor for the U.S. military, made him anathema to the student body. At the time, I opposed the boycott because of free speech issues.

Serendipitously, years later, in 1985, I found myself spending two days in a flooded airport with Huntington! He was then working with the United Nations' Brundtland Commission. Its main achievement was the publication of a report responsible for popularizing the term "sustainable development." We were wet and bedraggled, in the middle of a monsoon in Xishuangbanna, in China's Yunnan province, bordering Myanmar and Laos. I was visiting what later became the Xishuangbanna Biosphere Reserve. It was a perfect opportunity to reminisce—but not to heal the disagreements. At least the monsoon created an environment of mutual respect (which lasted until the weather broke!).

Returning to my time at Sussex, the dean of biology, John Maynard Smith, had created an intellectual environment that helped students navigate through the tumult of the times. My studies introduced me to the work of scientists such as Paul Ehrlich, Lynn Margulis, and James Lovelock, showing me how the perspectives of science can lead to vision and activism. This led me to make a personal commitment to transformation, to creating the world we want to live in. For me, this meant not trying to change the system from within, but instead creating an alternative outside its embrace. Of course, such a feat is technically impossible, as all human endeavor and creativity, all art and science, are reflections of the culture that birthed them. That said, after many years my early naive perceptions have been confirmed: Everyone I have known who chose to work from within their system was changed/compromised/moderated/mainstreamed to the point that the only activism left was the language used.

I entered the field of medical herbalism in the 1970s. It was a different world: pre-Thatcher, pre-Reagan, pre-punk, Afghanistan was still a kingdom, there was no internet, no social media, no i- or e- anything! Interestingly, it was also before evidence-based medicine became a thing. Attitudes toward clinical herbal medicine by the mainstream ranged from a patronizing paternalism mansplaining how wrong herbalism was to aggressive condemnation of its dangers. The main criticism was that herbalism was based on tradition, not science, and therefore had no credible evidence. It was claimed that using alternatives such as herbalism stopped people from seeking real medicine, and as such was dangerous. Ironically, such statements were themselves not supported by any evidence.

My education, and the culture it served, told me that herbalism had been relegated to the compost heap of history. I was told that the traditional use of plant medicines was over in the U.K. (and, in fact, in all other "civilized" countries), with no living tradition. From behind my overeducated privileged blinkers, I did not conceive of looking for an herbalist to apprentice with and learn from. Instead, I studied to become a consultant medical herbalist. At the time this term described practitioners trained in both herbalism and medicine, sidestepping concerns about misleading the public and avoiding perceptions of practicing medicine without a license. My intense education in the safe and effective use of plant medicines in health care was probably the best available anywhere in the Western world during those days of herbal drought.

The word *phytotherapy* had not yet entered the English lexicon, and its science-based attitudes and perspectives were still on the student fringes. The older members of the National Institute of Medical Herbalists were practitioners of the old-school American physiomedical and eclectic herbalism through the filter of the industrial world of the North of England. In their terms, I suppose it was "no-nonsense herbalism." Little attention was given to concerns that might illuminate holistic treatments; the major focus lay on the plethora of diagnostic, materia medica, and formulation issues that enable individualizing prescriptions. I am deeply thankful for this authentic training in Victorian clinical herbalism. In a way it was a very allopathic approach. English medical herbalism was empirical—we were using herbs to treat illness based on generations of observation of outcomes and formulation criteria originally developed in nineteenth-century America but further developed in twentieth-century Britain. There were minimal philosophical underpinnings, unlike the fundamentally holistic systems of Asia, like traditional Chinese medicine and ayurveda.

My exploration of herbalism beyond the clinic soon highlighted the limitations of this medical worldview.

Classical Greek had a diversity of terms for herbalists of various kinds. *Rhizotomoi*, "root cutters," gave rise to *rhizomatist*, a name used to describe the modern herbalist. Sellers of herbal medicines were the *pharmacopuloi*, whereas ointments came from the *unguentii*. All of these were stored in *apothecae*, or warehouses, where they were sold by the druggist, or *apothecarius* (Kremers, Sonnedecker, Urdang 1986, 17).

Rather than *rhizomatist*, perhaps a better descriptive name for an herbalist today would be *radicle*. This term traditionally refers to the growing tip of the root, which is perhaps one of the strongest forces in the natural world—just think of little shepherd's purse cracking sidewalks! *Radicle* as a name for an herbalist pairs nicely with its homonym, *radical*, one of whose definitions in Webster's dictionary is "favoring extreme changes in existing views, habits, conditions, or institutions."

Consider this example of radicle herbalism: how herbal health care leads to cultural change. It's change on a small scale, but what more can we really hope for? I had a practice in the city of Port Talbot, South Wales, which at the time was at the heart of post-industrial-revolution dereliction. Here one could find vast hills of mine and factory waste that were so polluted with heavy metals, such as cadmium and lead, that no plants could grow. Researchers at what was then called University College of Swansea developed grasses and other plants with the ability to absorb the metals without being poisoned. The hills are now green in the spring, with flowers in the summer, but no animals are allowed to graze on the grass because of toxic levels of heavy metals.

The Port Talbot Steelworks, one of the biggest steel production plants in the world, combines with other heavy industry and an urban motorway to gift the city with air pollution—a 2005 study ranked it the worst in Wales, measuring particulate pollution at 31 micrograms per cubic meter (BBC News 2005). The World Health Organization's recommended limit is 15 micrograms per cubic meter. Of course, there are more kinds of pollution in the air of Port Talbot than particulate emissions, but it gives a sense of magnitude of the problem. (Nevertheless, as the site of the Baked Bean Museum of Excellence, Port Talbot may still be worth a visit!)

I had a patient from Port Talbot with black lung disease (pneumoconiosis), or scarring of lung tissue caused by inhalation of coal dust, making it difficult to breathe. It's an occupational ailment common in miners. He was in his early fifties, unable to work, and receiving disability pension. At our first meeting, I could hear his distressed breathing as he struggled to climb the few stairs into my building. Over the next few months his breathing capacity improved, but I know of no successful herbal treatment for curing this debilitating condition. There are, however, herbal approaches to easing the symptoms, yet his therapy and its benefits are not the point here.

After some months, he started talking about his grandson, who was finishing up school and looking for work, but the only job available was "going down the mines." My patient obviously didn't want his grandson getting black lung. When next we talked, he had been mulling over the coal mine and its waste, his improving breathing, and the herbs that were helping him—herbs that were no longer growing locally because of the pollution.

Through the very personal experience of plants helping him, it seems, his perspective changed. Coal caused his illness, and mining waste destroyed the soil on which the herbs that helped him grew. He wanted to see changes, and the situation had become personal. His self-interest had started him along the path of becoming an eco-activist.

A few years later I saw him on TV debating a representative of the U.K. National Coal Board. Every time the politician tried to minimize the problem of air pollution and industrial dereliction, my patient would start wheezing. He always won the argument!

An appropriate perspective for a modern herbalist would be to be both radicle and radical. Question authority, and especially herbal authority. This does not mean denying facts or simply disagreeing, but always assess validity. Deconstruct the plethora of belief systems that underlie many of the assumptions of modern herbalism. Be aware of the way meta-context subtly conditions perception and vision. However (and isn't there always a however?), do not mistake the herb industry as being synonymous with the herb community. On good days, I see the industry as facilitating herbalism; on bad days, it's a parasite sucking on herbalism's lifeblood.

For my part, I am not celebrating the dominant culture embracing herbalism. I am instead affirming the fundamental nature of grassroots resistance: a timeless expression of the green in the face of humanity's tendency to pillage the natural world's resources. Nevertheless, celebrating the planetary perspectives emerging in human consciousness is not to deny the reality of the fascist last gasp. The toxicity of the resurgent extreme right cannot be overemphasized. But herbal practitioners treat the signs and symptoms of toxicity every day!

This book is at heart one herbalist's affirmation of the power of grassroots herbalism—an affirmation of the ancient, multicultural, scientific, yet magical planetary family we are rooted in. As we keep nurturing the herbs, we keep being nurtured by them. Herbalism cannot, on its own, heal the world; it will not ride in to save us in our time of need. It is not special and is no more unique than any other path. But perhaps, if all those multitudinous paths converge in the same direction, if they point the rising wave of human self-interest in the direction of planetary consciousness, we might stand a chance.

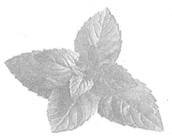

INTRODUCTION
Embrace of the Green

The word *herb* means different things to different people, with definitions varying according to areas of interest and personal bias. What, then, is herbalism? Just saying that it is the study of herbs begs the question. The lack of clarity reflects the changing fortunes of herbalism in English-speaking cultures over the centuries. At one time herbalism was an honorable profession that laid foundations for modem medicine, botany, pharmacy, perfumery, and chemistry, but as these fields developed and our culture's infatuation with technology and reductionism took over, herbalism was relegated to the history books or pleasantly quaint country crafts. This left *herb* as a word with a variety of uses but lacking a cultural core. As herbalism develops afresh in what has been called the "herbal renaissance," it is time for this little word to be reclaimed.

The *Shorter Oxford English Dictionary*, fourth edition, gives the primary definition of *herb* as follows: "A plant of which the stem does not become woody or persistent (as in a shrub or tree), but remains more or less soft and succulent, and dies down to the ground (or entirely) after flowering." A second definition says that the term *herb* is "applied to plants of which the leaves or stem and leaves are used for food or medicine, or in some way for their scent or flavor."

Botany views herbs as nonwoody plants—that is, plants without woody lignin fibers. The science of ecology has a very specific definition; in descriptions of complex communities such as forests, herbs are

1

plants that are less than twelve inches high that live their life cycles in the "herb layer." But this would suggest that even trees and shrubs such as sarsaparilla and cramp bark, though long known as sources of healing remedies, are not herbs.

In the various branches of medicine, the word *herb* usually implies plants that are sources of healing remedies, whether in their "crude" form or as extracts of physiologically active chemicals. But this can lead to only physiologically potent plants being recognized as herbs, ignoring the gentle tonic remedies.

From the perspective of an herbalist, an herb is any plant material that may be used in the field of health and wholeness. The term may refer to an herb in the strictly botanical sense with a remedy such as horehound, or it may refer to a part of a plant as in the flowers of calendula, the heartwood of the lignum vitae tree, the seeds of chasteberry, or the roots of echinacea.

One general definition that is often given states that an herb is "any useful plant." However, what plant is not useful? Indeed, it could be argued that poison oak is exceptionally useful as it encourages people to avoid certain places on the land. This plant has its ecological niche on disturbed soil, deterring animals with its extremely irritating oil. Up until the recent past, disturbed ground would have been mainly the result of landslides and earthquakes. Today it is largely the result of human activity. Poison oak acts as an ecological vulnerary (wound healer), deterring human irritants and the damage they cause. The wholeness of the environment is vital for individual human health, implying that all plants in our environment have a medicinal role to play in planetary terms.

If the holistic context is taken in its broadest sense, then an herb is a plant in relationship with humanity, and herbalism becomes the study and exploration of the interaction between humanity and the plant kingdom. Such a stance highlights the range and depth of human dependence on plants. This relationship is at the core of agriculture, forestry, carpentry, construction, clothing, medicine, and so on.

Herbalism is common to all peoples and cultures of the world. This shared experience of alleviating suffering through the use of plant medicines bridges cultural divides, religious differences, and racial conflicts. A relationship exists between each culture and its plant environment, in which the herbalist plays a pivotal role. Herbalism is more than knowledge about healing plants—it encompasses all of the experience and wisdom born of this relationship between humanity and plants.

Herbalism is reappearing in many varied ways, but they all can be seen as part of a broader and deeper embrace of the "green." Most manifestations are clearly positive contributions to the quality of the lives of people, health care, and so on. Others are part of the seemingly endless battle between belief systems conveniently called the culture wars. Some aspects of the herbal renaissance are becoming relevant to mainstays of the dominant culture, while others might be characterized as resistance to the dominant culture. However, many expressions of this movement are simply manifestations of capitalism at work. The implications and meanings are contextual, entirely dependent on philosophical or political context, in the same way that a single economic statistic might be interpreted as a sign of the end of capitalist oppression or as evidence of an attractive profit stream.

How do all these conceptual changes affect herbalists? The scientific developments and paradigm massaging in play raise many questions and issues, but to quote the Talking Heads from their song "Once in a Lifetime": same as it ever was!

Although our modality has developed and grown in the past forty years, the practice of herbalism, in all its multifaceted manifestations, has not changed in any fundamental way. There has been no essential change in the clinical realities, in protocol development, or in the criteria for herb selection. My limited observation of traditional Chinese medicine and ayurvedic practice seems to show similar affirmation of their traditions. Of course, there have been remarkable strides in clinical competence and expertise, educational excellence, and the availability of medicines of the highest quality and reliability.

It is in the world of mainstream medicine that insights about herbs and traditional herbal approaches are bringing about profound changes.

We are dealing with new regulatory environments, as well as the expectations of evidence-driven medicine.

This book offers a brief retrospective on herbalism, and writing it has either illuminated some insights or confirmed my biases—the reader must decide. My main conclusions go beyond the new science, as the path of the herbalist is so much more than a scientific one! Throughout the world and across all of history, humanity has based its many approaches to health care on the use of medicinal plants. This has led to a wonderful mosaic of healing traditions that reflect the rich diversity of human culture that gave them birth. This diversity mirrors the many differences of environment, history, and human needs around the world. However, this diversity can also obfuscate the shared botany, the fundamental similarity of humanity, and the aspiration to alleviate suffering.

Recognition of the value of herbal medicine has come from various directions. Crucial among them has been the people's positive response to good herbal medicine because it works. As explored in the following chapters, a solid scientific basis has been demonstrated from which valid therapeutics have been developed. This is an expression of ecology as healing, with a progression from the soil to the home medicine chest, the clinic, the laboratory, and eventually recognition by the World Health Organization.

The richness of the herbal traditions of the world reflects the diversity of human cultures, healing traditions, spiritualities, and belief systems combined with the cornucopia of herb diversity. This means herbalism is a place where the realities of nature get mixed with human hearts and minds, so it can get messy. The very success of herbalism necessitates a road map. Let's start with a look at the structure of this book.

Chapter 1 introduces ideas and concepts that provide a language and map for all that follows. This material, developed in more depth later, offers an overview of the wide range and culturally diverse nature of herbalism. We'll look at the origins of herbalism from an Earth-centered perspective, using the lens of ecology and evolution rather than the usual cultural, medical, or botanical viewpoints. We'll borrow the concept of deep time to explore the paleolithic evidence for herbalism and the origin of herbal traditional ecological knowledge (TEK). More context comes from a brief review of herbal history from the perspective of social activism, focusing on a few examples.

Chapter 2 attempts to put the use of medicinal plants in the context of relevant therapeutic systems from around the world. The abundance of culturally and regionally specific traditional healing approaches, or folk medicines, is most immediately insightful. We'll also examine the ancient and inherently holistic systems of ayurveda (from India) and traditional Chinese medicine in comparison to the Western biomedical model, which is now the dominant system worldwide.

Chapter 3 examines the nomenclature of herbalism, beginning with the not-so-simple question of what is meant by the word *herb*! Much disambiguation and context are needed to justify the relevance of herbal perspectives. In a culture that is so ambivalent about herbs and herbalism, finding herb-related words with multiple meanings, used in multiple ways to say different things, can be perplexing. Can sense be made of the confusion of names in folk herbalism? It is not simply words that need defining, but numbers, too, that need measuring and evaluation. Further, in the process of making sense of herbal diversity, a daunting question is posed: How many herbs are there?

Chapter 4 is a brief exploration of the new science that has revolutionized the perspectives through which herbalism can be seen. For once, the use of the phrase *paradigm shift* is actually appropriate. So an old herbalist looks at the new science, with a brief introduction to some of the transformative changes in the life sciences subsequent to the Human Genome Project. This chapter examines systems biology and "omics" sciences (especially metabolomics), which are greatly relevant to the use of herbs, as well as network pharmacology, which tantalizingly promises the marriage of omics, systems biology, and herbal complexities.

Chapter 5 explores the concepts of bio- and chemodiversity.

Invoking the ideas *ecological theater* and *evolutionary play*, it presents the diversity of herbal secondary metabolites as being ecologically and therapeutically related. The core concept is that secondary metabolites facilitate ecological interfaces. This insight resonates on all levels— therapeutically, personally, socially, and politically. The chapter examines the roles played by secondary metabolites in ecology, revealing interactions of all kinds and discussing a few particular examples, such as terpenes and sesquiterpene lactones, in detail. Integrating all of these concepts, we finish by looking at the planetary ecology of aroma.

The same secondary metabolites that do so much for plants and their environment are involved in many kinds of interactions within cells. **Chapter 6** considers the pharmacology of secondary metabolites, using herbal examples to illustrate the multitude of ways in which they affect metabolism, making both the therapeutic and the coevolutionary implications clear. This chapter also examines the foundational role of medicinal plants in both historical and modern drug discovery.

Chapter 7 takes us in a different direction, examining the role of herbalism in the face of the existential crisis now threatening humanity. Itself a human endeavor, herbalism is as distorted and in need of becoming "woke" as all else in this culture. As an example, we examine the herb industry in North America, which fulfills the irreplaceable role of supplying herbs to the ever-growing herbal marketplace. But rather than affirming herbal tradition, it has commodified medicinal plants and introduced herbalists to the joys of the supply chain. Today, the freedom of choice we encounter when buying an herbal product is not actually freedom—it's corporate bread and circuses. So maybe there are parallels between the tulip mania of the seventeenth century and the marketplace explosion of CBD and marijuana today.

In the face of this trend, modern herbalism must work to turn back to the people rather than professional elitism or marketplace commerce. Herbalism is now present in our culture, having come out of the garden shed (instead of the closet), and is now playing an ever-increasing and more visible role. Nevertheless, the questions need to be asked: in what role, in what reality, and to what end? Medicinal plants do not come with an ideology or belief system, and we can look to the embrace of herbalism and natural medicine by the Nazis in the mid-1900s for cautionary lessons in these times of reawakening fascism.

Chapter 8 is a reality check. Any attempt to identify a role for herbalism in the future needs to be based in clarity and honesty about the nature of what humanity is facing. It gets dark. The planetary crisis of climate change and subsequent environmental change lead to global catastrophic risks. The nature of the Anthropocene, with climate tipping points and biodiversity loss, threatens not only societal collapse but also an unprecedented ravaging of Gaia. Any response to what is now called the polycrisis needs to be on a planetary scale, but there is little meaningful change from governments, corporations, or elites. Meanwhile, the UN is calling for an end to the "orgy of destruction," and the worldwide science community has issued warning after warning, publishing the data, the facts, the predictable outcomes.

Chapter 9 poses the question: What is a simple herbalist to do? This last chapter is an affirmation of simplicity and the gift of viriditas— greening power—in the form of herbalism. Leaving the disaster speak behind, how might herbalism, with its roots in deep time, help us reach a future? At its heart, herbalism is a repository of ancient TEK. It facilitates the empowerment of people through grassroots medicine, letting botany cross cultural divides. This chapter explores some of herbalism's many contributions to community resilience. The use of herbs in emergency response, for example, can be seen as human-scale mitigation and resilience building. Emphasizing the importance of an herbal first aid kit, the chapter discusses how to create one and offers a brief guide to what types of herbal medicines might be useful, how to make them, and how to select herbs to get to know. It finishes by reviewing the self-created, self-directed education field of the modern herb world in North America and various examples of successful community herbalism, which are an ever-growing and increasingly appreciated presence in many places and often find a role in supporting underserved communities.

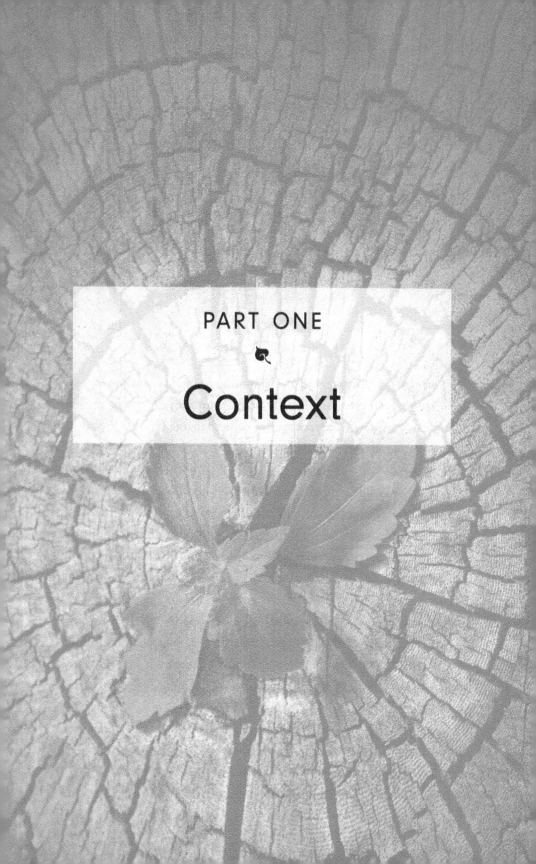

PART ONE

Context

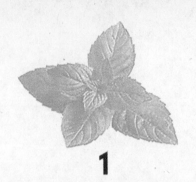

1

The Deep Roots of Modern Herbalism

Human perceptions and understandings change and evolve over time, yet herbalism is still here! Was a dead Greek military doctor, Dioscorides, really the father of herbalism? If so, who was the mother (let alone the midwife)?

The use of herbs in healing did not start with the names history has given us—Ashurbanipal, Shen Nung, Dioscorides, or others. While these names are central to any historical perspective on how herbalism developed over time, and we will reference them later, these towering figures from the mainstream narrative are potentially a distraction from the perspectives of an Earth-centered history. They wrote it down but didn't create it. History as perceived by the dominant culture is distorted by written records because the only people who wrote down records were those with the opportunity (the time, tools, and education) to write. This may be obvious, but for there to have been something to write about, it would have to have been experienced first. So can we trace the origins of herbalism?

If we go beyond the classical tomes and look toward evidence from nature, a very different picture appears out of the past. Rather than the historical perspective usually applied in discussions of herbalism, we'll examine an ecological/evolutionary context. From this vantage point, connections and correlations that are otherwise obscure become clear, revealing the deep roots of modern herbalism—roots in the natural world and a shared human experience.

The biological reality of comprehensive integration among organisms (plants, fungi, bacteria, and animals) has been a characteristic of life for billions of years. For example, the land was colonized by the ancestors of modern land plants about 500 to 470 million years ago. Land plants first appear in the fossil record in the mid-Ordovician period (about 470 million years ago), and by the middle of the Devonian period (about 390 million years ago), many of the features recognized in land plants today were present, including roots and leaves. As we shall explore later, cooperative interactions with fungi were fundamental to this development (Heckman et al. 2018).

The concept of deep time was originally applied to the vastness of geologic time but is also used in archaeology. Paleoarchaeologists study fossils ranging from fifteen million to ten thousand years ago, exploring human evolution and adaptation to the environment in the past few million years. However, finding evidence of medicine use is challenging because plant remains rarely survive, and evidence showing the deliberate medicinal use of plants is even more rare. *This means looking for links and correlations.* A good example is assessing the evidence from remains showing long-term survival following disease or physical trauma.

Consider skeletal remains from 1.7 million years ago, from the subspecies *Homo erectus*, found in Georgia. These remains show that this individual lived for several years despite having lost all their teeth to periodontal disease, which can cause brain abscesses as well as cardiovascular disease. To quote prehistory archaeologist Karen Hardy, "The survival of this individual may have been down to extraordinary luck, but the use of antibacterial plants may well have saved them" (Hardy 2021).

Consider also the seven-thousand-year-old skeleton of a person who survived having their left arm amputated, as demonstrated by healed scars. In fact, recovery from amputation was fairly common in prehistory. Postsurgical recovery generally requires prevention or treatment of infection, suggesting that our ancestors had a deep knowledge and skill in the use of medicinal plants.

These and many other examples imply a high level of plant-based medicinal knowledge extending deep into human evolutionary time. The increasing evidence for self-medication in animals suggests a shared evolutionary behavior that stretches back to a time before humans.

Plants Used as Medicines by Animals

The science of zoopharmacognosy studies animal self-medication—that is, how animals select and use plants, soils, and insects for healing. Chimpanzees, for example, exhibit a great degree of botanical knowledge, including where to find specific plants, when and how much to eat, the correct part of a plant to use, and, if necessary, how to prepare it. Of the two hundred to three hundred species of plants they regularly eat, at least thirty-six are medicinal (Hardy 2021).

Some of the best-studied self-medication practices in animals are the way chimpanzees deal with intestinal parasites. In one example from the 1980s, researchers in Africa observed a sick female chimp build a nest in a tree. She then sought out bitter leaf (*Vernonia amygdalina*), a plant chimps do not normally eat, broke off branches, and sucked juice from the tips. This plant is poisonous in high dosages but at low dosages is rapidly effective for digestive problems caused by parasites. The chimp rested for a day in the nest she had built for the occasion. She then seemed to feel better and left to catch up with her troop (Velasquez-Manoff 2017).

Bitter leaf contains a number of constituents that are quite effective against parasites. Their efficacy was reflected in the rapid decline in the number of parasites found in the chimp's stool, a decrease of more than 90 percent in one day. The herb could easily kill a chimp, and so the dosage is crucial, implying great skill in using the right amount that was almost (but not!) dangerous but still killed the parasites.

Another example comes from chimps' use of *Aspilia*, a distant relative of daisy. When chimps eat plant leaves, they generally stuff the leaves into their mouths as fast as they can pull them off the plants and then chew them rapidly. They treat *Aspilia* leaves differently, though. A chimp will carefully close its lips over an *Aspilia* leaf—sometimes pausing for a few seconds—and often reject it without even pulling it off the branch. When a leaf meets with its approval, the chimp rolls the leaf around in its mouth, swallowing it whole before selecting the next one (Fowler, Koutsioni, and Sommer 2007).

Chimpanzees don't normally eat *Aspilia* leaves, but when experiencing abdominal distress they seek it out. Examination of the chimps' feces found that the whole-swallowed leaves remained intact and were accompanied by expelled worms. In one feces sample, twenty worms were found, along with fifty undigested *Aspilia* leaves. The mechanism appears to be the presence of stiff hairs on the leaves. When swallowed whole, rather than being chewed up, the leaves retain their rough, hairy surface, which is thought to help physically extract worms from their intestines. *Aspilia* is also widely used for human medicine in Africa. Local Tongwe people make a tea of the leaves to treat a number of things, including stomach disorders caused by worms.

If parasites cause chimps to self-medicate to alleviate the distress of the symptoms, what about other animals? There is an ever-expanding list of self-medicating animals. Goats in the eastern Mediterranean regularly consume resin from the mastic tree, which has strong antiparasitic effects. In Greece, that same resin is known as the "tears of Chios," being traditionally produced as "tears," or droplets, on the island of Chios (Soulaidopoulos et al. 2022).

African elephants have been observed traveling out of their usual feeding area to eat a particular species of tree. The leaves and bark of this tree are known to induce uterine contractions; they are occasionally used by pregnant Kenyan women, in tea, to induce labor or abortion (Huffman 2022). Similar behavior has been observed with Asian elephants in Thailand (Greene et al. 2020).

Orangutans in Borneo have been observed using an herb to soothe inflammation. The apes chew leaves of *Dracaena cantleyi* to create a white lather, which they rub onto their bodies. These leaves contain a constituent that inhibits the production of inflammatory cytokines, substances that can aggravate inflammation in the joints and muscles. People on the same Indonesian island are known to use this plant for the same purpose (Morrogh-Bernard et al. 2017). Dracaenas are popular houseplants. The name derives from the Greek *drakaina*, "female dragon," due to a red gumlike resin in the stems of some dracaenas that was likened to dragon's blood. This resin has been used medicinally for generations.

Female muriqui monkeys in Brazil prepare themselves for the mating period by eating the leaves of three plants that they ignore the rest of the time. Two of the plants contain phytoestrogens, compounds similar in effect to the hormone estrogen. The third plant contains a constituent that, once consumed, is converted to progesterone, increasing a monkey's chance of becoming pregnant (de Carvalho, Ferrari, and Strier 2004).

Many animals show self-anointing behavior, getting rid of parasites by rubbing plants on their skin or lining their nests with them. In Costa Rica, white-faced capuchin monkeys harvest the fruits of specific species of citrus and rub the pulp and juice into their fur. In Panama, white-nosed coatis take the aromatic resin from freshly scraped bark of a tree related to myrrh and vigorously rub it into their fur to kill parasites such as fleas, ticks, and lice, as well as biting insects such as mosquitoes. This resin is antimicrobial and antiparasitic (Wainwright 2002, 135–39).

All of this provides a broad evolutionary backdrop and context within which our ancestral use of medicinal plants sits comfortably. From an evolutionary perspective, it is inconceivable that our human ancestors would have abandoned this very advantageous behavior, and given the constant battle against parasites and pathogens of all types that animals (including humans) experience, it is unlikely they would have survived without the ability to treat some of them.

The very widespread use of medicinal plants among animals supports the perspective that this behavior has a long evolutionary pathway. The extent of animal self-medication implies it is behavior that is evolutionarily beneficial. We can infer that it was practiced by our direct hominin ancestors as an essential mechanism for survival and that it formed a part of the human evolutionary package.

This suggests that self-medication among Paleolithic populations is an evolutionary adaptation, inherited from our animal past, that developed and expanded throughout prehistory (Hardy 2019). At some point, knowledge of the medicinal and psychotropic properties of plants merged and developed into what today is called shamanism.

Plants Used for Intoxication by Animals

The desire to experience an altered state of consciousness is seen in every culture and civilization worldwide. One way to achieve this is through the use of psychoactive plants, and as with plants used for medicine, there are many examples of animals seeking out specific plants for their psychoactive effects.

Cats Using Catnip

Perhaps the most familiar example of animals using intoxicants is that of cats and catnip. Ailurophiles (from the Greek *ailouros*, meaning cat, and *-phile*, meaning lover) are familiar with cats' enthusiasm for catnip. The felines eat its flowers and roll around on the leaves and stems. In a matter of minutes they show signs of intoxication, such as rolling, licking, rubbing themselves, stretching, jumping, and sleepiness. They may even hallucinate while under the influence of catnip, as many exhibit hunting behavior even when no prey is present (Tucker and Tucker 1988).

Deer Eating Psychedelic Mushrooms

Reindeer, also known as caribou, actively seek out psychedelic fly agaric (*Amanita muscaria*) mushrooms frozen beneath winter snow. People who have seen them after they've eaten the fungi describe the deer showing "drunken" behavior, including aimless running, head twitching, and noisemaking. The metabolic process of detoxifying muscimol, the hallucinogen in fly agaric, by the liver of caribou generates the safer and stronger psychoactive psilocybin, which is removed from the body in the urine. This makes the urine actively psychoactive. The psilocybin will, in fact, readily affect people who drink caribou urine, so that in Siberia and

Lapland this became a custom. This phenomenon might be the origin of Rudolph the red-nosed reindeer. The story of Rudolph and his flying friends originates in Siberia, where the mushroom grows in abundance and knowledge of its effects on reindeer would be well-known.

This all suggests a general direction for our herbalistic roots—word-of-mouth transmission of a collective body of plant knowledge and skills that developed over the deep time of the Paleolithic human experience. This in turn evolved (as humanity evolved culturally) from the herb usage of other primates and thus from the collective oneness of biology.

Signs of the use of medicinal plants extend as deeply into the past as archaeology has looked. Researchers have found evidence of the developing use of medicinal plants that may have contributed to health and vitality deep into the Lower Paleolithic (Hardy 2019). And although the dominant culture sees the relationship between people and plants as one of domination and domestication, modern scholarship envisions a very different relationship, one of coevolution between plants and humans (Allaby et al. 2015).

Paleolithic Man and
Traditional Ecological Knowledge

The various regional, culturally diverse forms of traditional herbalism today represent the relict survival of our deep evolutionary inheritance, a very ancient knowledge system known today as traditional ecological knowledge (TEK). In one modern definition, TEK is "a cumulative body of knowledge, practice, and belief evolving by adaptive processes and handed down through generations by cultural transmission about the relationship of living beings (including humans) with one another and with their environment" (Reyes-García et al. 2014).

TEK developed during the Paleolithic as humans established and expanded their understanding of their environment, most probably, at times, by observing and copying the behavior of other animals. The ability to identify and use appropriate plants would have been a basic component of the ecological knowledge that underpinned Paleolithic life. In this way, TEK provides context for how knowledge about the medicinal and health-providing properties of plants has endured over very long timescales and is part of the enduring heritage of our hunter-gatherer past.

Until recently, TEK was seen as a vestige of the past that was bound to disappear with economic development. Yet it is now clear that substantial pockets of TEK persist in many cultural and geographic areas, even those that have been "modernized." These pockets of social-ecological memory comprise places or activities that have stored and transmitted through time specific knowledge and experience. These biocultural "refugia" of traditional knowledge show that some TEK systems can be resilient to modernization and themselves contribute to sustaining biodiversity and ecosystem vitality, building resilience in the face of global change. Use and knowledge of herbs and herbalism is a prime example. In the face of industrial capitalist medicine, herbal knowledge from humanity's evolutionary deep time is not only remembered but clinically proven!

A growing number of archaeological sites are providing evidence for the diverse uses of plants by Neanderthals (Shipley and Kindscher 2016). This has contributed to an appreciation of the cultural and ecological sophistication of Neanderthals, illuminating the importance of plants in their diet and in their medicinal and ritual traditions. We will examine here two examples. In the first, we have evidence of a purely biological nature: the use of medicinal plants. In the second, we have a cultural expression: the burial of an herbalist.

Teeth to Feces

Extracts from dental remains of a Neanderthal found in El Sidrón cave, in northern Spain, found high levels of yarrow and chamomile. Both are well-known medicinal herbs with no purely nutritional properties. This suggests that the Neanderthal ingested the plants for their medicinal properties rather than as food (Shipley and Kindscher 2016).

The need for essential nutrients alone does not explain the numerous plant species found in some Paleolithic sites. The presence of a wide range of plants with important medicinal compounds at such sites suggests their use both to sustain health and to treat common problems such as intestinal pathogens. Their medicinal profiles are likely to have been a significant factor in their selection for use and the broad-spectrum approach to plant exploitation throughout the Paleolithic.

When plant remains are found at an archaeological site, plants that are known to be edible are generally assumed to have been consumed. The same assumption can be applied to plants with therapeutic effects; we can only assume they were used for those effects. Numerous plant remains have been found at Paleolithic and Neolithic archaeological sites. Around half of the plants that can be identified have medicinal properties. Some plants are both edible and medicinal, but some, as in the case of the Neanderthal remains discussed above, are nonedible and/or non-nutritional, allowing us to surmise that they were collected specifically to treat ailments (Hardy 2019). The most common medicinal benefits of the plants examined are their antibacterial, antioxidant, antimicrobial, and astringent properties. That is, these plants would be best suited to treating ailments such as diarrhea and dysentery as well as wounds.

At all sites, plants that have both edible and medicinal properties predominate; however, over time, there is a clear positive trend reflecting an increase in the diversity of plants with medicinal properties. This suggests an expanding knowledge and use of medicinal plants over time. The increasing proportion of plants that are both foods and medicines suggests that the use of these was a successful strategy that expanded and developed over time. Inclusion of plants with medicinal compounds in the diet would provide a broad underlying resistance to pathogens, while deliberate selection of curative plants to deal with specific ailments is in line with evidence from a range of animals.

In Brazil, similar conclusions were drawn from studies of pollen found in coprolites (Miranda Chaves and Reinhard 2006). The word *coprolite* comes from the Greek *kopros lithos*, meaning "dung stone," and refers to fossilized feces. Pollen analysis of eight-thousand-year-old coprolites clearly shows that our ancestors from this time period were consuming medicinal plants. Identifying the plants allows speculation about the uses they were being put to; the coprolites contained pollen traces from plants similar to those used today to treat lice, parasites, worms, arthritis, respiratory problems, dysentery, wounds, and pain, among other conditions.

Shanidar

Shanidar Cave in Kurdistan provides the earliest clear evidence of people using plants for medicine rather than food. Here, the skeleton of a Neanderthal man, approximately thirty to forty-five years old and dating back sixty thousand to eighty thousand years, was found buried in a partial fetal position. Pollen from soil samples gathered around the body suggests that entire flowering plants were buried with him. The plants are ones with known pharmacological activities, including bachelor's button, cornflower, hollyhock, horsetail, ragwort, and yarrow, all of which known to be diuretics, astringents, and anti-inflammatories. Based on when these flowers bloom, the authors of the study wrote, "one may assume that the placement of the Neanderthal man . . . on a bed of flowers occurred more than 50,000 years ago between the end of May and the beginning of July." They speculate that this man "was not only a very important man, a leader, but also may have been a kind of medicine man or shaman in his group" (Shipley and Kindscher 2016).

A History of Herbalism

History is written by the victors, as the saying goes, and so any historical perspective is by its nature biased, whether culturally, politically, ideologically, or personally. This means that any history of herbalism is a reflection of the cultural worldview through which it is perceived. What follows is my own brief personal perspective on the history and historiography of herbalism. It emphasizes what might be called "people's herbalism" or the medicine of the oppressed—somewhat anathema to the mainstream.

Herbal history has many facets, reflecting the diversity of topics embraced by the term *herbalism*. For example, focusing on a particular herb would illuminate the plant's evolutionary and ecological history, history of human use, history of commerce, science and drug development, regulatory history, and current legal status. Such a focus would also explore the medical uses of the herb, showing how they may have changed over time and across cultures. This would illuminate how the different world traditions (e.g., traditional Chinese medicine, ayurveda, biomedicalism) view the herb in their unique paradigms.

However, a history of herbalism would also explore humanity's relationship with herbs, including how they were and are used, prepared, and cultivated, as well as their cultural role and their position in "professionalized" herbalism.

The written history of herbalism is predominantly that of the dominant culture's use of herbs, a history that leads to seeing herbs as raw materials for drug development and thus fodder for capitalism and European colonialism. We'll explore a number of these issues in later chapters, but here we'll focus on examples of people's herbalism—how people in diverse cultures have related to herbalism, as opposed to the writings of experts on how best to use herbs in the medical practice of the day.

If we are to explore people's herbalism, a natural starting place is indigenous herbalism. The dominant culture—the elite of academia, industry, and government—has tended to ignore the wisdom, insights, knowledge, and skill of the indigenous people of the world, including their relationship with plants. But who are the indigenous? Originally meaning something naturally occurring in a particular region or environment, such as indigenous plants or indigenous culture, *indigenous* also often refers to the earliest people of a region and specifically one that was colonized. Of course, in the face of the global marketplace, we are all the indigenous.

Historiography looks at the way history is written, focusing not on the events of the past, but on the changing interpretations of those events. Today, many historians are focusing on the history of dissent and the experiences of minorities, the disadvantaged, and the displaced. We'll do the same, employing a coevolutionary context—looking at the coevolution of plants and humans—and emphasizing ecological biochemistry, throughout this book. This puts the human history of herbalism in a more illuminating perspective.

Ancient Foundational Texts from around the World

The importance of herbalism in human history is highlighted by the fact that some of the earliest written texts known concern medical practices and the use of plants as medicine. (Though, as noted earlier, examining the history of herbalism based on written texts means drawing primarily from the perspective of the educated, literate elite.) Several important foundational texts from the world's herbal traditions demonstrate a deep understanding of plants, medicine, and pharmacy. These ancient documents include examples from Egypt, Mesopotamia, India, China, Greece, and the Middle East (Hardy 2021).

Egypt

A number of ancient Egyptian papyri, from between 2000 and 1500 BCE, contain extensive information about medicinal plants, their use, and their preparation, suggesting a materia medica of more than 160 herbs (Frey 1985). The Ebers papyrus, dating to around 1550 BCE, is considered to be the most important and extensive of surviving records of Egyptian medicine. Rich in herbal knowledge, the papyrus is a 110-page scroll, about twenty meters long, containing formulas and descriptions of a range of remedies. In addition to its extensive materia medica, the papyrus contains chapters on health care generalities and treatment protocols for heart conditions, depression and dementia, contraception, intestinal diseases, parasites, and eye and skin problems.

Mesopotamia

Hundreds of thousands of medical texts from ancient Mesopotamia, dating from the third millennium BCE, were written mostly on clay tablets in cuneiform. Because clay tablets are more durable than papyrus rolls, more original medical records survived from Mesopotamia than from Greece or Rome. The largest surviving medical text is the "Treatise of Medical Diagnosis and Prognoses," which dates to around 1600 BCE; it contains a summation of several centuries of Mesopotamian medical knowledge.

Many of the surviving Mesopotamian texts were found in what's called the "Library of Ashurbanipal," a collection of more than thirty thousand clay tablets and fragments from the time of the Assyrian king Ashurbanipal, who ruled from 669 to 631 BCE. The collection was discovered in the ruins of the city of Nineveh (in what is now northern Iraq), once the capital of the Assyrian empire.

India

Originally shared as an oral tradition, the principles of ayurveda were first recorded more than five thousand years ago in the four sacred Sanskrit texts called the Vedas: the *Rig Veda* (3000–2500 BCE), *Yajur Veda*, *Sama Veda*, and *Atharva Veda* (1200–1000 BCE). Ayurveda is rooted in the three foundational texts called the Brihattrayi, which describe the basic theories and practices from which the modern practice has evolved. They are the *Charaka Samhita* (600 BCE), *Sushruta Samhita* (500 BCE), and *Ashtanga Hridayam Samhita* (400–500 CE).

China

Traditional Chinese medicine has a written history dating back to the early Zhou dynasty (ca. 1050–256 BCE), and its evolution into an extraordinary system of healing was well documented in ancient medical texts. The most famous four classics are Inner Canon of the Yellow Emperor (Huang Di Nei Jing, ca. 26 BCE), Yellow Emperor's Canon of Eighty-One Difficult Issues (Nan Jing, ca. 106 CE), Treatise on Cold Damage Disorders (Shang Han Lun, ca. 206 CE), and Shennong's Materia Medica (Shen Nong Ben Cao Jing, ca. 220 CE). In total, the ancient literature of China records more than a hundred thousand herbal recipes.

Greece

Herbs were a cornerstone of treatment in the medicine of classical Greece. Hippocrates (460–377 BCE) was among the first to consider illness a natural rather than a supernatural phenomenon, and in his writings, he discussed herbs within the context of a wonderfully holistic perspective.

First-century Greek physician Dioscorides wrote *De Materia Medica*, a five-volume medical text listing about six hundred herbs and focusing on the preparation, properties, and testing of drugs. This work had an astonishing influence on Western medicine, becoming the principle pharmacological reference in Europe and the Middle East until the seventeenth century.

Roman physician Galen wrote an enormous body of medical texts over his lifetime (129–201 CE). Galen's works came to symbolize Greek medicine to the medical scholars of Europe for the next fifteen centuries. His theories became dogma throughout the West.

Middle East

In the Middle East, the practice of medicine thrived from about 500 to 1500 CE, integrating concepts from Greek, Roman, Mesopotamian, and Persian medicine. Islamic medicine preserved, systematized, and developed the medical knowledge of Greece and Rome, translating writings from Greek or Latin into Arabic. Later, in the twelfth century, Western scholars rediscovered the principles of ancient Greek medicine by translating Islamic texts back into Latin. As they were elsewhere, plants were the basis of medicines in the Islamic tradition, with about 250 species being core remedies (Saad, Azaizeh, and Said 2005).

Dissenter Herbalists

History is replete with people who questioned the status quo or dissented from the accepted norms. The history of medicine is no different: Since the very beginnings of the medical "academy," there have been doctors and herbalists who were dissenters and iconoclasts.

As Western cultures became increasingly centralized and dogmatic, the simple, wild-sourced, community-based nature of herbal medicine didn't fit in. Herbalists often found themselves opposed to policies enforced under the authority of religious, medical, legal, governmental, or scientific power.

The examples that follow show the interface between dissenter herbalists and the control they deviated from. We'll begin with the viriditas-illumined herbalist Hildegard of Bingen, who, throughout her life, experienced immense challenges posed by the Church of Rome. For the seventeenth-century English herbalist Nicholas Culpeper, the societal dissent that characterized the English Civil War gave birth to his complete dissention from the social role of pharmacy. Culpeper wrote his famous work, *The Complete Herbal*, as an overt act of rebellion by democratizing access to herbal medicine. In North America, in the early years after the founding of the United States, the work of Samuel Thomson was as much part of the spirit of dissent of his time as it was part of herbal history.

Hildegard of Bingen

Hildegard of Bingen (1098–1179 CE) was a mystic and Benedictine abbess whose vision and spirituality filled her writings, music, and art. She wrote extensively on herbalism and medicine as well as cosmology, theology, and natural history.

For Hildegard, the Divine manifested itself in nature, leading to the concept of *viriditas*, meaning the divine force of nature or "greening power" of God. As this divine power is transferred from the plant to human, it becomes an expression of viriditas. If the life-affirming and harmonizing attributes of viriditas are blocked, Hildegard believed, the barrenness and dryness of *ariditas* occur. Physical disease is the manifestation of such inhibition. Hildegard's healing protocols and herbal recommendations are profoundly holistic, recognizing the broadest perspectives of healing and not just symptom relief. Carefully selected and appropriately prepared herbs were used in conjunction with dietary and lifestyle guidance.

Hildegard's vision often transcended that of the Church. She saw the Divine as female as much as male and considered both essential for wholeness. Resisting the patriarchal church hierarchy, she pushed the established boundaries for women.

Her willingness to question long-established ideas, dissenting from the norms of tradition, was seen not only in her herbalism but in all aspects of her work. Late in her life, the Archbishop of Mainz ordered Hildegard to exhume the body of a young man who had been buried on sacred ground despite having been excommunicated. Hildegard refused, as the man had sought absolution and received grace, and she told the archbishop that only his own stubbornness and pride prevented him from recognizing this. The archbishop then excommunicated her and the rest of her convent, with the sisters being forbidden to receive Communion or to sing. The excommunication was lifted only when the archbishop died, shortly before Hildegard's own death in 1179.

The wisdom of her words and the transformative beauty of her art and music have remarkable effects even today. Viriditas is expressed in every word, note, and brush stroke. In the book's conclusion, we'll return to Hildegard and the relevance of her insights to the modern day.

Nicholas Culpeper

One of Britain's best-known herbalists, Nicholas Culpeper (1616–1654), is another exemplar of the activist herbalist. Culpeper vehemently asserted that medical treatment should not be limited to the privileged. To champion the needs of the people who could afford neither the services of a doctor nor the expensive medicines they prescribed, he wrote and published *The Complete Herbal*, a comprehensive listing of English medicinal herbs and their uses, in 1653. It became an instant bestseller and appeared in many subsequent editions.

But this was not Culpeper's first act of rebellion. In 1618, during a time of strict control by the medical authorities, the Royal College of Physicians (RCP) had published the *Pharmacopoeia Londinensis*, which was backed up by a royal proclamation from King James I. It included an officially sanctioned list of all known medical substances (chemical, herbal, or animal), their effects, and directions on their use. No one was allowed to make, sell, or dispense any substance for medical purposes if it did not appear in the *Pharmacopoeia Londinensis*. Thus the practice of medicine and pharmacy was, in effect, controlled by the RCP. The RCP had the power to inspect apothecary shops in London and regularly destroyed any drugs being sold that the college deemed unsuitable. There are numerous accounts of apothecaries (pharmacists) being fined or imprisoned for not complying with the RCP's edicts.

In 1649 Culpeper published an English translation of the pharmacopoeia, under the title *The London Dispensatory*, making the Latin names of substances and methods of preparation readily accessible to lay readers, while also adding explanations and new (unapproved) formulations they could use. His work was roundly condemned by the Royal College of Physicians.

The revolutionary act of Culpeper's translation was making such knowledge available to all, not just apothecaries and physicians. He gave away the trade secrets!

Samuel Thomson

Medicine in North America has a rich tradition of dissent. Samuel Thomson (1769–1843) developed what might be described as "backwoods naturopathy" by blending the use of herbs and sweat baths. His system was partially a reactionary counterpoint to the heroic medicine of the day, which was based on the use of bleeding, mercury, and arsenic. The Thomsonian system used energetic ideas of heat and cold, positioning heat as life-supporting and cold as life-threatening. Substances that stimulated heat in the body, such as diaphoretic herbs, were widely used, while substances that introduced cold into the body, such as mercury, aconite, and opium, were avoided.

Thomson had a strong belief in an individual's ability and right to self-treat and firmly believed that the practice of healing should remain with laypeople. Underpinning his adamant belief that his system of healing should be practiced only by householders was his strong aversion to the medical education and practice of his day. The animosity engendered by his stance was the beginning of the adversarial relationship between herbalists and MDs that was so characteristic of the United States throughout the twentieth century.

The Unknown Herbalists

To be an herbalist in the English-speaking world during the twentieth century was, almost by definition, to be a dissenter. Herbalism was seen as an avocation whose time was past, antiquated, irrelevant, or at best charmingly quaint. With no meaningful niche in the modern world, the only reasonable response was to dissent from that world, creating alternatives, and so become part of the healing of the culture. Misquoting the aphorism, herbalists didn't ask for permission because what they were doing did not need forgiveness.

Immediately we are faced with the reality of what might be called the "unknown herbalists," the people who used, collected, and grew medicinal plants without making a big deal of it. They didn't write books, teach, or become influencers. They helped their family and neighbors with simple natural medicine, but their contribution to the health and well-being of society has not been recognized or quantified by sociologists or epidemiologists. It may be that this grassroots herbalism created a health care safety net for many people who were priced out of the U.S. medical system.

The rediscovery of this often invisible role played by herbalists is actively underway. As an example of such rekindled interest in culturally specific herbalism, consider the impressive research into the herbal traditions of Eastern European Jews recently published in *Ashkenazi Herbalism* by Deatra Cohen and Adam Siegel. The depth and quality of research undertaken by the authors is especially remarkable considering the impact of the Holocaust on all aspects of Ashkenazi life in Eastern Europe. The Nazi ravages decimated not only Jewish herbalists (along with everyone else) but the culture and records of the communities they served.

John Christopher

Dr. John Christopher (1909–1983), a naturopath and herbalist, was one of the last exponents of therapeutic approaches rooted in the pioneering herbalism of Samuel Thomson. In 1953, Dr. Christopher set up the School of Natural Healing, which is still operating today, to train herbalists, and many would consider his book *School of Natural Healing* to be essential reading for Western herbalists. He had a strong belief that herbs were a healing gift from God, and so he was willing to practice herbal medicine quite openly, leading to confrontations with the American Medical Association and even occasional imprisonment for practicing medicine without a license. His dissent was a major contribution to the birth of the herbal renaissance.

Herbal Educators

The modern herbal movement has created a unique array of educational options and pathways for practicing healing modalities, often in the face of cultural derision and regulatory oppression. This can be seen in what until recently was a uniquely North American phenomenon of grassroot herb schools—that is, educational pathways created by herbalists for herbalists, not mainstream schools identifying a new topic with an untapped student stream.

An excellent example of all that is positive in modern dissenter herbalism can be seen in the Vermont Center for Integrative Herbalism. Conceived, created, and run by grassroots activist herbalists, the center declares (on its website): "We are . . . dedicated to providing a range of healthcare resources grounded in Nature. Our work brings clinical herbalism to community practice through the weaving of science, spirit and grassroots activism." Their commitment to this vision led to a recognition that herbal education was part of their healing work: "We provide one of the nation's most extensive clinical training opportunities in herbal medicine, rooted in deep connection with the plants and place." They have now taken this educational effort further by collaborating with Goddard College to develop a program enabling their students to apply their herb school learning toward credits in a tailored program of study at Goddard.

For more on herbal education, see page 168.

Pivotal Moments in Herbal History

The timeless earth-centered nature of herbalism does not insulate it from the culture it is part of. The history of herbalism is always a component of a culture's history, and vice versa. For example, some events in Western history have been pivotal in the development of Western herbalism. Consider the following.

The Burning Times

Any study of the history of European herbal traditions would highlight the Burning Times of the Middle Ages. The main accusations of the great medieval witch hunts were primarily three: every conceivable sexual crime against men; organizing and conspiring against authority; and having magical powers affecting health—of harming, but also of healing. So-called "witches" were often charged specifically with possessing medical and obstetrical skills.

The *Malleus Maleficarum* (1486), usually translated as "Hammer of Witches," is the best known treatise on witchcraft. It states, "No one does more harm to the Catholic Church than midwives" (Kramer and Sprenger 2007). Puritan theologian William Perkins (1558–1602) had this to say:

> For this must always be remembered, as a conclusion, that by witches we understand not those only which kill and torment, but all Diviners, Charmers, Jugglers, all Wizards, commonly called wise men and wise women . . . and in the same number we reckon all good Witches, which do no hurt, but good, which do not spoil and destroy, but save and deliver. . . . It were a thousand times better for the land if all Witches, but especially the blessing Witch, might suffer death. (Perkins 1618, chapter 7, section IV; spelling updated)

Based on records of the Inquisition from around Europe, not just women but also many men were condemned as witches. In Iceland, more than 90 percent of accused witches were men, and in early Muscovy, about 75 to 80 percent were men (Rhodes 2020).

The medieval attack on herbal healers could be seen as a reaction to the power exerted by healers, which threatened Church and State. The greater their power to heal, the less they were dependent on God and the Church. Their cures interfered with the will of God, authorities said, and were achieved with the help of the Devil, making the cure itself evil. There was no problem in distinguishing God's cures from the Devil's, for obviously the Lord would work through priests and doctors rather than through peasants.

There is no written record of the wise women and green men of this time, the herbalists who kept their tradition going and, we hope, were doing their best to ease suffering. The history of the people's herbalism has yet to be written and will call for the skills of a historiographer to follow the hints and clues.

This pivotal period reinforced the patriarchal hierarchy that became the organizational structure of medicine in Europe. The herbalist, midwife, and healer (whether woman or man) came to be seen as an outsider whose moral, legal, and scientific raison d'être was culturally dubious at best, and anathema at worse.

Chartism and Founding of the NAMH

In Britain, the early nineteenth century was an era of social ferment. The year 1819 saw the Peterloo Massacre in Manchester, in which cavalry charged into a crowd of around sixty thousand people who had gathered to demand the reform of parliamentary representation. Voting rights were finally enacted in 1832, but only for property owners. Further political reform was needed, and the Chartists were the response, working to gain political rights for the working class. Chartism is named after the 1838 People's Charter, a listing of the aims of the movement, which included a vote for all men, a secret ballot, no property qualification, payment for MPs, and electoral districts of equal size. (Such concerns are all still relevant today in these times of gerrymandering.)

The Chartists' political agitations led to a rising tide of populism in Britain, including in the field of medicine. Taking a cue from the

Thomsonian practices of the United States, physiomedicalism took root, partly as a rejection of the medical practices of the day, which included the use of mercury and bloodletting. The physiomedicalists practiced an herbalism imbued with a vitalist grasp of health, building a sophisticated system of clinical practice and marrying the evolving science of the day with herbal medicine.

The modern incarnation of public herbalism in the U.K. can be traced to the 1864 founding of the National Association of Medical Herbalists (NAMH), the precursor of today's National Institute of Medical Herbalists. The NAMH's goals, as described by Richard Lawrence Hool in a 1922 publication for the organization, included "the diffusion of a knowledge of the Therapeutic properties of Plants" and "the development of the Herbal Practice of Medicine and of Herbal Pharmacy." This would be achieved by "utilizing the principles of Physio-Medicalism" (Hool 1922). In other words, under the NAMH, professionalization of herbalism would rely on such populist concepts as dispersing knowledge widely, encouraging the use of natural remedies rather than only sanctioned apothecary medicines, and acknowledging the innate vital intelligence that animates and heals every living organism.

1883 U.S. Dispensatory

The fifteenth edition of the *U.S. Dispensatory* (or *The Dispensatory of the United States of America*, as it's officially known), published in 1883, can be seen as a glaring representation of official medicine's historical bias against "folk remedies." We can look, for example, at the well-known medicinal plant skullcap (*Scutellaria lateriflora*), which has played a central role in North American folk medicine for hundreds of years, with ancient Indigenous American use. It was included in the U.S. pharmacopoeia until the 1920s as a relaxing, tonic nervine. It was widely used by U.S. eclectic physicians and European phytotherapists as a tonic, relaxing nervine and antispasmodic. It is currently a mainstay of modern British clinical phytotherapy, focusing on its anxiolytic properties and ability to ameliorate symptoms of premenstrual syndrome. The *British Herbal Pharmacopoeia* highlights skullcap's anticonvulsive and sedative actions, indicating its use in nervous tension states and epilepsy. Research has found that flavonoids in the herb bind to GABA (gamma-aminobutyric acid) receptors in neurons, thus having a relaxing effect (Wolfson and Hoffmann 2003). GABA is a major inhibitory neurotransmitter in the central nervous system. GABA receptors on nerve cells receive the chemical messages that help to inhibit or reduce nerve impulses. The flavonoids from skullcap bind to the same receptors as GABA and so mimic GABA's calming effects. The nonprofit American Herbal Pharmacopoeia has published a comprehensive monograph on skullcap, covering botany, microscopy, phytochemistry, pharmacology, therapeutics, and U.S. as well as international regulations (Upton 2009).

The calming effects of skullcap are not subtle; they are very real, while at the same time not overly intense. The important point is that they are genuine and readily experienced.

However, that is not evident in the supposedly objective entry in the 1883 *U.S. Dispensatory:*

> To the senses skullcap does not indicate, by any peculiar taste or smell, the possession of medicinal virtues. It is even destitute of the aromatic properties which are found in many of the labiate plants. When taken internally, it produces no very obvious effects, and probably is of no remedial value, although at one time it was esteemed as a remedy in hydrophobia. It is also used by some practitioners as a nervine in neuralgic and convulsive affections, chorea, delirium tremens, and nervous exhaustion from fatigue or over-excitement. (Wood et al. 1883)

The writer's conclusions are not based on science or clinical observation but suggest a professional bias when seen in the context of the intellectual ferment science experienced at the end of the nineteenth century. Plants were used extensively throughout medicine. However, eclectic doctors and pharmacists were much more open to medicinal plants that were indigenous to North America. From the mainstream European perspective, skullcap was simply a weed to be ignored. If the great medical schools of Europe ignored the herb, it was of no value, according to the "experts" in charge of such things as compiling guidelines for dispensing medications.

The Flexner Report

In 1910 a report on medical education in North America was published, with momentous effects. The author, Abraham Flexner, not only examined the state of medical education but made a number of recommendations. These included reforms such as improving educational standards, establishing partnerships between schools and hospitals to facilitate clinical training, and closing schools that did not meet these standards. Today the publication of the Flexner Report, as it is known, is seen as the beginning of modern medicine by the mainstream, but as almost the death knell of health care freedom by others. Among other criteria, it graded medical schools on the quality of their science education and how well they adhered to the protocols of mainstream science in their teaching and research. The report transformed medical education, establishing the biomedical model, with its solidly science-based worldview, as the de facto standard of medical training (Stahnisch and Verhoef 2012).

The Flexner Report achieved the establishment of a standardized medical curriculum across U.S. universities. It led to a reduction in the number of poorly trained physicians while at the same time increasing the quality of new physicians. However, these improvements came at a cost. Just to begin, so many medical schools were rated of poor quality that the total number of schools offering medical education dropped from 155 to 31. Additionally, Flexner considered non-science-based approaches to medicine as quackery, so medical schools offering training in modalities of herbal medicine were told to drop these courses or lose accreditation. The report advocated for closing most programs in homeopathy, naturopathy, eclectic therapy, physiomedicalism, osteopathy, and chiropractic. A few schools resisted for a time, but eventually all complied with the report. The last eclectic medical school, in Cincinnati, closed in 1939.

For the next hundred-plus years after the publication of the Flexner

Report, the various modalities that embrace natural medicine had to take a backseat to biomedicalism. Physicians became specialists in crisis care management, though often failing their communities with respect to general health and well-being. The biomedical model works well when it comes to acute pain, sickness, or injury, but it is not well set up to foster health. It is now evident that defining health as the absence of disease has been a major contributing factor in the modern world's increased incidence of chronic disease, and that a holistic approach is critical in achieving health and preventing disease.

The Flexner Report's radical restructuring of formal medical education, perhaps ironically, created the educationally bereft environment that led to the flowering of the herbal renaissance—that is, herbalism from the ground up, not the ivory tower down.

Herbal Renaissance

By the 1960s and '70s, traditional herbalism was largely absent from the dominant culture, having been seemingly relegated to the ever-growing pile of quaint "folkways" discarded by scientific triumphalism. Of course, herbalism was alive and well outside the mainstream in some Indigenous American, immigrant, and other communities, but it was invisible in mainstream U.S. education and media. However, something unexpected was brewing. The '60s were a time of self-empowerment, of creating a new world, of people (especially the young) questioning what they were being told and what governments and elite institutions were doing. The tumult was not only to be seen in all aspects of society but carried many people to a rediscovery of nature and inner life. It was as if the spirit of nature had burst through the gloom of fifty years of world wars, the deep trauma of the Great Depression, and the insanity of the Cold War and the "mutually assured destruction" of nuclear confrontation. Around the world, people felt this "sunlight," often for the first time.

In much of the Western world, this conceptual transformation led to the birth of what came to be called hippie counterculture. One aspect of this eruption of joy and celebration was a rediscovery of herbalism and TEK—the wisdom of the old ways. This led inexorably to a natural approach to health care, especially herbal medicine and the personal and cultural resilience it offers. By the 1970s, herbalism's reemergence had spread well beyond the radical fringe into the culture in general—a process that is ongoing to this day. As the flower power generation learned, herbalism had never gone away but simply went underground to stay safe!

Herbalism's new popularity was famously described as an "herbal renaissance" by herbalist Steven Foster in a 1993 book bearing that phrase as its title. The herbal renaissance is much more than herbs becoming easily available or the marketplace discovering a profit stream from herbal products. It is, in essence, our culture rediscovering that it has a place in nature.

In the twenty-first century, herbalism has matured into a vibrant presence, developing in a number of ways. Science has recognized medicinal plants as an exciting area of study, ranging from pure research into constituents and pharmacology to practical applications. Of crucial importance has been the investigation of herbs and herbalism in the real world of health care, from the ethnobotany of folk medicine to evidence-based assessments of clinical outcomes.

In 1994 the U.S. Congress passed the Dietary Supplement Health and Education Act (DSHEA), a statute defining and setting up a regulatory framework for dietary supplements, including herbal remedies. The DSHEA opened up a new profit stream for capitalism, facilitating the development of a dynamic marketplace for herbal products and meteoric growth in the industry. Unfortunately, this trend occasionally takes the form of illusory "miracle cures," herbs with useful properties that are marketed with false claims promising unobtainable outcomes. From the 1990s, when echinacea was touted as a replacement for antibiotics and St. John's wort was proclaimed the answer to depression, to today, when CBD (cannabidiol, from hemp) is sold as a cure for everything, the attempts to market tradition as the latest trend are embarrassing.

On the other hand, a quieter, deeper, and truly significant movement has developed, bringing its breath of fresh green air to everything it touches. Hildegard's vision of viriditas, the healing power of the green, is actively at work transforming individual lives, communities, and entire cultures, contributing greatly to healing humanity's fractured relationship with Earth. This is an actual grassroots movement—a flowering of interest in all aspects of herbalism arising directly from the people, not a social media phenomena generated by "influencers."

Practitioners of herbal medicine are privileged to be carriers of a tradition whose origins cannot be traced. We live in a time when traditional knowledge has been demeaned and devalued. Practitioners have little if any legislative support, receive their training in exceedingly modest educational facilities, and have no access to the public hospital system, limited access to diagnostic services, and a questionable professional status. Despite this, the practice of herbal medicine continues to remain a vital and enduring source of satisfaction both for those who would carry the tradition through mastery of its methods and for those who seek out the services of knowledgeable practitioners.

2

Using Herbs in the Context
of a Therapeutic System

Plant treatments are at the core of many diverse medical systems of the world, from traditional Chinese medicine (TCM) and Indian ayurveda to Western therapies like herbalism, homeopathy, aromatherapy, and Bach flower remedies. Many drugs currently used in orthodox medicine were derived from plant constituents or are actual plant products.

As affirmed by the World Health Organization (WHO), all medicine is "modern" as long as it is directed toward the goal of providing health care. The essential differences among these various systems of medicine are related to their cultural contexts, rather than their goals, techniques, or effects. The WHO recognizes that all traditions have value and that any particular worldview is limited, as it operates only within the belief system of one tradition. Thus, the view of reality from the cloisters of a Western medical school is as limited and limiting as that from a shaman's hut in West Africa. All perspectives have value in any worldwide approach to enhancing health for all.

This diversity is an expression of the intimate relationship between people, their culture, and the plants they live with. Every human culture is filled with the bounty of this relationship in its arts, in its cuisine, and of course in the herbal basis of its practice of medicine. The manner in which herbs have informed healing and health care are many and varied.

Among the herbal healing systems in current use, some depend upon traditional knowledge, while others work within the framework of an existing philosophical system. Systems based on the folk traditions of the world vary according to the tradition used. Those that work within the framework of an existing system differ depending on the philosophy at their core. Philosophical contexts include the profoundly holistic systems of Asia as well as the Western medical approach, which is based on what has been called the biomedical model.

Traditional Healing Systems

The traditional or folk use of herbal remedies is familiar to everyone in some form or another. This is the way in which information about herbs has been passed from generation to generation. Folk wisdom is of inestimable value and relevance. Generations of accrued experience and insight are not to be taken lightly. The bulk of the world's health care is still based on the traditional use of local herbal remedies. The relevance of this worldwide folk use is recognized by the WHO and promoted through its Global Centre for Traditional Medicine. Every culture of the world has its own herbal tradition, which may be either a thriving aspect of modern life or a more or less moribund historical memory.

However, as fundamentally valuable as traditional folk knowledge is, it has limits within modern holistic herbal practice. An application of herbal remedies that relates specific plants to specific diseases or symptoms is little more than what we might call "organic therapy." Simply using remedies for symptomatic relief ignores all the insights of holistic medicine.

Philosophical Systems

The way in which herbs and herbal medicine as well as health and wholeness relate to a culture's worldview is fundamentally important. At the deepest level, there is a clear differentiation between systems that are part of a holistic/spiritual worldview (such as TCM and ayurveda) and those that are firmly based in the biomedical model (dominant culture medicine).

Phytotherapy offers the most value to holistic medicine when used within the context of a coherent philosophical system. Such systems work with conceptual models for understanding what a human being is and what a disease process is. Each system's concept of health and human wholeness must be seen as a subset of the paradigm held by that culture about the nature of the world itself.

Such paradigms are reflected in the holistic medical systems of China and India as well as in the strictly biomedical model of Western medicine. Traditional Chinese medicine, ayurveda from the Vedic tradition of India, and unani from the world of Islam represent the best-known examples of philosophical systems that are still thriving in the face of the reductionist imperative of Western medicine.

The techniques of any medical system are an expression of its ideas and theories. These, in turn, arise as specific developments in the philosophy of the culture concerned. Thus, traditional Chinese medicine represents an application to medicine of a Confucian or Taoist worldview. Similarly, ayurveda is an expression of the philosophical perspectives that come from Hindu experience and spirituality.

Western Herbal Medicine

Despite regional variations, herbalism is increasingly popular in Europe and North America, and in some countries it is widely practiced by orthodox medical practitioners as well as by qualified herbalists. The Western tradition has a long history, with the roots of its practice found in the writings of the Greek physicians, such as Hippocrates and Dioscorides, as well as later in the works of the Romans, such as Galen. As is the case with other systems, maintenance of health is fundamental to the practice of Western herbal traditions.

Indigenous North American Herbal Medicine

Traditional Indigenous American medicine (or, as it's sometimes known in Canada, Aboriginal traditional medicine) refers to the various systems of healing used by Indigenous American nations. While they have similarities, there are often significant differences between the practices or herbal traditions of different tribes. In general, Indigenous American medicine is holistically linked to philosophy, religion, and spirituality, and its treatments aim to balance the physical, emotional, mental, and spiritual components of a person.

Traditional Chinese Medicine (TCM)

TCM is based on an energetic worldview, and a central insight is expressed in the concept of yin and yang, two opposing yet complementary forces that are said to shape the world and all life. Harmony between these two forces supports health; an imbalance between them can result in disease. Their energetic interaction is facilitated by qi, vital energy that circulates in the body through a system of pathways called meridians. The ultimate goal of TCM is to balance the yin and yang in a person's life by promoting the natural harmony and flow of qi.

TCM recognizes five elements (fire, earth, wood, metal, and water) to symbolically represent all phenomena and explain the functioning of the body and how it changes during disease. Resting on these principles is the whole array of TCM theory and application.

The concept of synergy is intrinsic in TCM philosophy. As in other herbally based therapeutic systems, the herbs in TCM formulations are blended to enhance the bioavailability of active components, promote therapeutic effects, and/or reduce toxicity. Much attention has been given to the scientific proof and clinical validation of these herbal formulations, requiring a rigorous approach that includes chemical standardization, biological assays, animal models, and clinical trials. Such Western methodologies can fail to take into consideration the synergistic potential of the formulations, both among their own constituents and with the human body.

Ayurvedic Medicine

Ayurveda is the dominant herbal tradition of South Asia and arguably the oldest system of healing in the world, with records going back five thousand years, predating Chinese medicine. The system is widely practiced in Europe and increasingly present in North America.

Ayurveda is based on concepts of universal interconnectedness—relationships among people and their world. All things in the universe, living and nonliving, are said to be joined together; health represents the mind and body being in harmony and interaction with the universe flowing naturally. Thus, disease indicates a person is out of harmony with the universe. Disruptions can be physical, emotional, spiritual, or a combination of these.

The ayurvedic idea of constitution (prakriti) refers to general health and the ability to resist and recover from diseases. Prakriti is characterized by the interplay of the three doshas (vata, pitta, and kapha), which, together control the activities of the body. Vata combines the elements of ether and air, controlling basic body processes such as cell division, heart rate, breathing, and discharge of waste as well as the mind. Pitta represents the elements of fire and water, which control hormones and the digestive system. Kapha combines the elements of water and earth, which help maintain strength and immunity and control growth.

Unani Medicine

Unani is a traditional system of medicine on the Indian subcontinent and in the Arabian world. The impact of Greek medicine is evident, with Hippocrates considered to be the first unani physician. However, this system got established under the patronage of Persian and Arab empires and came to India around the middle of the fourteenth century. Health is seen as a state of equilibrium in the four humors (blood, phlegm, yellow bile, and black bile), in which the functions of the body are normal in accordance to its own temperament (cold, hot, wet, dry) and the environment.

Homeopathy and Herbal Medicine

Homeopathy and herbal medicine are conflated by everyone other than their respective practitioners! There is a common misconception that these two healing modalities are the same because they both employ plants. Indeed, herbs are used in both approaches, but in radically divergent ways that reflect differences in philosophy and therapeutic technique.

Homeopathy was developed in Germany by Samuel Hahnemann more than two hundred years ago, although it has roots in the writings of Hippocrates. It's based on three theories. First is the concept that "like cures like"—that a disease can be cured by a substance that produces similar symptoms in healthy people. Second is the law of minimum dose, which states that the lower the dose, the greater its efficacy. Third is the principle of the single remedy, based on the idea that a homeopathic remedy has been proved by itself, producing its own unique drug picture, and that remedy is matched (prescribed) to the sick person having a similar picture. The results, when observed, are uncluttered by the confusion of effects that might be produced if more than one medicine were given at the same time.

Homeopathic remedies are made in a unique way. Substances become remedies through the very specific process of sequential dilution and succussion (a hard pounding or shaking). The more the dose of the remedy is reduced, the more its potency is enhanced. This is why the homeopathic process of dilution is known as *potentiation*. The dilution of one part of the active remedy in ten parts of the solvent (usually water) is known as a potency of 1X. A dilution of one part remedy in one hundred parts solvent is 2X, and so on, up to a dilution of 200X. Remedies in the range of up to 30X are considered low potencies, while those of 200X or above are considered high potencies.

An herb used homeopathically is prescribed in dilution to treat symptom pictures that supposedly match the symptoms that would be caused by a full dose of the herb. This idea is easy to understand with a poisonous herb such as belladonna. However, it is problematic with remedies shared by homeopathy and herbalism. An example is the homeopathic remedy Cimicifuga, based on the plant known as black cohosh to the herbalist. Both the homeopathic remedy and the herb are used to treat painful menstruation with upper back pain. In other words, the symptom picture for homeopathic Cimicifuga is also *treated* by black cohosh, not *caused* by black cohosh, which would appear to contradict the core idea behind homeopathy. The same holds true for a number of other herbs, including some well-known home remedies: They are used by both homeopathy and traditional herbal medicine for similar purposes. Consider calendula for wound healing, chamomile for easing teething pain, witch hazel for healing hemorrhoids and varicose veins, and boneset for alleviating stiffness and bone pain associated with flu symptoms.

The value of homeopathy in health care is not in question here, but its use of plants is in no way "herbal." A selection of one or the other therapeutic modality should be based upon attraction to the philosophical context, recognizing that there is little to no real sharing of the principles of botanical medicine.

The Biomedical Model

The National Library of Medicine describes the biomedical model of medicine as focusing on purely biological factors and in its purest form would even exclude psychological, environmental, and social influences (Wade and Halligan 2004). This is still the dominant way for health care professionals to diagnose and treat pathologies in most countries. According to the biomedical model, good health is the freedom from pain, disease, or defect. It focuses on physical processes that affect health, such as the biochemistry, physiology, and pathology of a condition. It does not account for social or psychological factors that could have a role in the illness. In this model, each illness has one underlying cause, and once that cause is removed, the patient will be healthy again. The focus is on objective tests rather than the subjective feelings or history of the patient.

The term *allopathic medicine* is often used to describe science-based modern medicine, although rarely by practitioners of the biomedical model themselves. The word was coined in 1810 by Samuel Hahnemann, of homeopathic fame, and was originally used by nineteenth-century homeopaths as a derogatory term for the heroic medicine of that era (1780–1850), which used extremely rigorous methods to "shock" the body back to health and balance the humors, including methods such as bloodletting, purging, vomiting, profuse sweating, blistering, and extensive use of mercury and other toxic heavy metals. One way of looking at it is that the patient needed to be a hero to survive! Heroic medicine fell out of favor in the mid-nineteenth century as gentler treatments and the idea of palliative treatment began to develop.

However, the World Health Organization in 2001 defined allopathic medicine as "the broad category of medical practice that is sometimes called Western medicine, biomedicine, evidence-based medicine, or modern medicine."

Today, the biomedical model is being slowly supplanted by integrative health care, which aims for well-coordinated care among different providers and institutions by bringing conventional and complementary approaches together to care for the whole person. Integrative care helps individuals, families, communities, and populations improve and restore their health in multiple interconnected domains—biological, behavioral, social, environmental—rather than just treating disease.

Modern naturopathic medicine marries the wisdom of nature with the rigors of modern science, with a focus on whole-person wellness through health promotion and disease prevention, while addressing the underlying cause of any ailment. The aim is to treat the individual by stimulating and supporting the body's inherent healing ability, to identify the root cause and address it as naturally and gently as possible, and to prevent illness whenever possible.

Within modern medicine, several modalities use herbs extensively, either as effective materia medica or as a component of holistic treatments—or both. Because of this range and diversity of users and prescribers of herbs, it is important to know the context.

Colpermin's Secret

From drug discovery and bioprospecting to digoxin and paclitaxel (Taxol), plants are deeply involved in modern medical life. Ipecac is perhaps the most widely available herbal medicine in North America (it is found in most first aid kits as an emergency emetic for poisonings). Of course, it is often difficult to see the presence of plants in modern medicine because the language describing drugs and medications is so different from the language of herbalism. The medicinal use of peppermint oil provides a good example.

Peppermint grows widely in Europe and North America. Medicinal use of this plant can be traced back to classical Greece, where peppermint leaf was used internally as a digestive aid and for management of gallbladder disease. Its aromatics were also inhaled, via steam, to relieve upper respiratory symptoms and cough. Extracts of peppermint are widely used as flavoring in many products, including toothpastes, mouthwashes, and over-the-counter gastrointestinal (GI) products. Menthol, a constituent extracted from peppermint, is a common ingredient in over-the-counter topical products used for respiratory congestion, headache, and muscle pain (Kligler and Chaudhary 2007).

Peppermint oil is antispasmodic by helping the muscle of the bowel wall to relax. Evidence strongly supports peppermint oil helping with symptoms of irritable bowel syndrome. It may also help with indigestion and prevent spasms in the GI tract caused by endoscopy or barium enema. The active constituents include menthol, menthone, cineole, and several other volatile oils (Blumenthal 2000). In vitro research shows peppermint oil to be effective in relaxing GI smooth muscle, possibly through an antagonistic effect on calcium channels in the gut (Hills and Aaronson 1991). However, peppermint oil also relaxes the lower esophageal sphincter, which can result in gastroesophageal reflux. Hence the use of enteric-coated formulations, which bypass the upper GI tract unmetabolized, thereby facilitating peppermint's effect in the lower GI tract without effects in the upper tract, easing IBS symptoms such as abdominal pain, bloating, and gas.

When these properties were recognized by gastroenterologists, they began to prescribe peppermint oil—but initially only in prescription form, for example, the trademarked medication known as Colpermin. Packaging and marketing of these effective medications gave no indication that they were of plant origin, much less that they derived from such a common, recognizable plant as peppermint. In fact, the FDA restricted imports of peppermint oil from Germany.

Today, enteric-coated capsules of peppermint oil—like Colpermin—
are available over the counter, without prescription, and are indicated
for the symptomatic treatment of painful bowel cramps and bloating in
irritable bowel syndrome.

Herbs are used in health care everywhere in the world, by all of the
diverse, culturally unique healing traditions humanity has created.
Systems such as ayurveda from southern Asia, traditional Chinese
medicine from China, kampo from Japan, and unani from the Islamic
world are all built around therapeutics that integrate herbal medicine
into profoundly holistic perceptions of the nature of health.

The systems just named earn some recognition from Western medicine because they have long written traditions and came from cultures
European imperialism has some begrudging respect for. However, the
use of herbs in Africa and South America has been largely ignored,
other than as possible new sources for pharmaceutical drugs. Similarly
ignored or devalued are the traditional herbalism of Europe, Russia, and
Turtle Island (North America).

The influence of medicinal plants is ubiquitous in mainstream
medicine, although it is often obscure. But once-fringe modalities in
Western health care are becoming more central, and their use of herbs
has been part of their success. Naturopathy is obviously the prime
example and can be cited as the primary expression of competent herbalism in accredited medicine in North America.

We'll discuss the pivotal role of plants in drug development, and
therefore pharmacological medicine, later, in chapter 6. Each medical specialty has its unique and relevant herbal materia medica. From
foxglove in cardiology to pain relief with morphine, heroin, and other
derivatives of the opium poppy to anesthetics derived from curare—all
highlight the ongoing and irreplaceable use of plants in medicine.

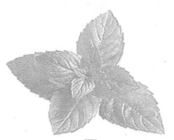

3

Names and Numbers: Defining Herbalism

How many herbs are there? But before that, how many plants are there, and how many of them are potentially medicinal? Such apparently simple questions are surprisingly difficult to answer. There are reasons why counting the number of living species is challenging. New species are constantly being identified, while others are becoming extinct. The 2023 *State of the World's Plants* report, from the Royal Botanic Gardens Kew, found that two thousand new plant species are discovered every year. However, the report also noted that one in five plant species is now threatened with extinction—and, unfortunately, extinction rates are increasing. Although extinction is a natural phenomenon, occurring at a "background" rate of about one to five species per year, the world is currently experiencing a rapid loss of species, at a rate estimated to be between a thousand and ten thousand times higher than the background rate (De Vos et al. 2015).

World Flora Online is a working online inventory of all known plant species, compiled through a partnership of various botanical gardens enacted as part of the U.N. Global Strategy for Plant Conservation. At the time of this writing in 2023, the database estimates that there are 383,054 species of plants, but that number is expected to eventually reach well over 400,000. The known species of vascular plants consist of 12,573 species of ferns, 1,311 species of gymnosperms (conifers, cycads, and allies), and 341,145 species of flowering plants (angiosperms).

How Many Herbs Are There?

Many countries publish pharmacopoeias, official government books providing precise and detailed descriptions of and tests to identify and assess the quality of plants used in commercial "herbal drugs." However, the number of plants in the various pharmacopoeias is a small percentage of the diversity of species used in traditional herbalism.

According to the International Union for Conservation of Nature and the World Wildlife Fund, between fifty thousand and eighty thousand species of flowering plants are used for medicinal purposes worldwide. This means that more than one-tenth of all known plants are used in health care.

The Medicinal Plant Names Services of the Royal Botanic Gardens Kew collated information on 28,187 species recorded as being used medicinally but found that only 4,478 are cited in regulatory publications (Allkin 2017). The low number of plant species covered by official pharmacopoeias reflects the globalization of a narrow range of species for use in herbal drugs.

For example, in the official Brazilian pharmacopoeia, the number of native Brazilian plant species decreased from 196 in the 1926 edition to 32 in 1959 and then to just 4 in 1977, before increasing again to 11 in 1996. The 2010 edition cites only 14 species native to Brazil. Similarly, in China, 10,000 to 11,250 species (around 34 percent of the native flora) have documented medicinal uses, but only 563 are cited in the Chinese pharmacopoeia. In India, some 7,500 plants are used medicinally, though only around 2,000 are used in ayurveda and listed in the Indian government's *Ayurvedic Pharmacopoeia of India* (Yao et al. 2023; Pan et al. 2014).

A fundamental problem with the attempt to quantify medicinal plant use is a matter of definitions and what counts as legitimate evidence. There is a difference between plants that can be shown to have pharmacological effects in the laboratory or clinic and those that have a recorded history of use in medicine.

So the answer to how many plant species are currently used as medicines depends on our perspective on medicine. If *medicine* in this context is taken to mean material recognized officially in approved pharmacopoeias, the number is clear and easy to find. However, if we apply a broader and more realistic definition and take into account the worldwide use of herbs in folk medicine, the number rises dramatically and is difficult to assess. But even this approach will identify only those species whose use as medicine has been recorded, which is obviously limited by how comprehensive the records are.

Making Sense of Herbal Diversity

The world is a cornucopia of plants with active effects in and on humans. From nutrition to healing and even poison, Earth's flora teems with human uses. This diverse herbal abundance arises in part thanks simply to the diversity of plants, which itself is often a characteristic of geographic and habitat regionality, compounded by the richness of multiculturalism that infuses herbalism. Faced with the vast array of potential herbal remedies, herbalists have developed ways of making sense of their options.

In formulating herbal medicines, the number of issues to consider can be daunting and include the consideration of various technicalities, such as the actions needed, body system affinities, plant chemistry, the inherent strength of the herb, medicine-making constraints, and sourcing limitations (and thus often cost). These calculations needn't be seen as confusing complexity but, rather, as manifestations of nature's abundance.

The multitargeted properties described for herbs can be a challenge for some to accept. How can one herb do so many apparently different things? Consider the range of properties of chamomile: It is a relaxing remedy that eases tension but also works as an anti-inflammatory that calms the inflammatory response in soft tissue, such as the stomach, the skin, and mucous membranes of the mouth and nose. At the same time, it makes a mild and pleasant beverage.

Herbs are not simple or singular. When it comes to their properties, the whole really is more than the sum of the parts. The bewilderingly diverse chemistry of the flora and the astonishing chemical richness of each herb provides the foundation for an array of properties.

Because of its chemical complexity, a single herb might produce a range of responses in the body. For example, chamomile contains several active components in its volatile oil, in addition to nonvolatile compounds and sesquiterpenes. This cornucopia of chemistry allows chamomile to act as an anti-inflammatory, antispasmodic, antimicrobial, and relaxing nervine all in one!

This highlights the different challenges posed depending on the perspective taken. If I may use an analogy: If you don't know your options, trying to find the correct herb for a particular situation is like desperately searching for an oasis in the desert, not knowing if such a place even exists. On the other hand, with some knowledge, your search is much more like looking for a healing spring in a deciduous wood. The challenge in this case becomes not the desperate search, simply hoping the answer exists, but rather avoiding sidetracks due to the richness of options.

Much pharmaceutical research has gone into analyzing the active constituents of herbs to find out how and why they work. However, a much older and far more relevant approach is to categorize herbs by the kinds of problems they can treat. In some cases the action is due to a specific chemical in the herb, while in other cases it might be due to an intricate, synergistic interaction between a number of the plant's constituents. It's always best to view the herb as a whole.

Let us look, as an example, at the categories of actions herbs might have when applied topically. In the context of first aid, the herbal actions most useful for topical application include:

- Anti-inflammatory
- Antimicrobial
- Antipruritic
- Astringent
- Rubefacient
- Vulnerary

Even within these limited categories, herbs offer a range of effects moderated by the method of application and the target of action. *Stellaria media* (chickweed), for example, is extremely effective for the relief of itching. The only itching for which it offers little relief is that due to jaundice. It is most effective in a nongreasy form, such as a bath, fomentation, poultice, lotion, or cream.

Let's dig a little deeper into the concept of the topical uses for herbs in first aid.

Anti-inflammatory Actions

Herbs that help the body combat inflammation are known as anti-inflammatory remedies. Mainstream medicine places much emphasis on chemicals that work to reduce symptoms of inflammation and ease suffering. However, symptom alleviation is not the best way to use herbal anti-inflammatories. They are safe to use for the relief of pain and discomfort but offer most when used in combination with other remedies to address the underlying problem.

There are many types of anti-inflammatory herbs, with varying chemistry and pharmacology. Attempts to classify these herbs by relative strength are not very helpful. It is far more useful in the therapeutic sense to group them in terms of the body system or tissue for which they are most appropriate or by their pharmacological mode of action. (This fascinating area of phytotherapy is beyond the remit of this current discussion, as our example at hand is first aid issues.)

Examples: Anti-inflammatory Herbs for Topical Use

Calendula	Horse chestnut
Chamomile	Irish moss
Chickweed	Meadowsweet
Comfrey	St. John's wort
Cranesbill	Yarrow

Antimicrobial Actions

Antimicrobial herbs help the body destroy or resist pathogenic microorganisms in some way. The action covers the whole gamut of microorganisms, including bacteria, fungi, and viruses. It would be a mistake to attempt an overarching generalization about mechanisms of action for herbal antimicrobials. The use of the term *antimicrobial* is a description of expected outcome rather than a specific process. Antimicrobial effects may be related to direct interactions with pathogens or mediated via the herb's interaction with the immune response. These herbs may also work through indirect actions by stimulating immune responses.

Examples: Antimicrobial Herbs for Topical Use

Calendula	Marjoram
Cayenne	Rosemary
Eucalyptus	Thyme
Garlic	Yarrow
Goldenseal	

Astringent Actions

The tightening of the tissue of the mouth caused by strong tea demonstrates the astringent action of the tea plant, *Camellia sinensis*. The astringency is due to a diverse group of complex chemicals, called tannins, that have some chemical and physical properties in common. The name *tannin* derives from the use of these constituents in the tanning industry. They have the effect of precipitating, or denaturing, protein molecules. This alteration of protein is how animal skin is turned into leather. In other words, astringents produce a kind of temporary leather coat on the surface of tissue. Because of this activity, astringents have several therapeutic benefits in that they reduce surface inflammation, creating a barrier against infection.

Examples: Astringent Herbs for Topical Use

Black tea	Shepherd's purse
Cranesbill	Witch hazel
Horse chestnut	Yarrow
Oak	

Rubefacient Actions

When applied to the skin, rubefacient herbs generate localized increase in blood flow. They are often used to ease the pain and swelling of arthritic joints. They produce redness of the skin by dilating the capillaries and thus increase blood circulation.

Examples: Rubefacient Herbs for Topical Use

Cayenne	Horseradish
Castor bean oil	Mustard seed
Garlic	

Vulnerary Actions

These remedies promote wound healing. While the term *vulnerary* is used mainly to describe herbs that heal skin lesions, the action is just as relevant for internal wounds, like stomach ulcers. That makes the large group of herbs with known vulnerary activity especially useful in the treatment of wounds, abrasions, and so on. The well-known vulneraries such as comfrey or calendula are excellent but not irreplaceable.

Examples: Vulnerary Herbs for Topical Use	
Aloe	Irish moss
Burdock	Marshmallow
Calendula	Slippery elm
Comfrey	Turmeric
Echinacea	Yarrow
Fenugreek	

Semantics and Misconceptions: The Confusion of Names

A review of 143 databases and publications found 415,180 unique names for plant-based medicines, and an average of 15 alternative names for each species (Allkin 2017)! In exploring the world through the lens of herbalism, we are immediately faced with a confusion of names and terminology. This reflects the diversity of languages, cultures, therapeutic systems, and scientific specialties to be found in the melting pot of herbalism.

What are we talking about? How do people of differing languages, cultures, and histories share and convey the incredible richness of their herbal traditions? As herbalism surfaces into the consciousness of the modern world, the need for a clear and unambiguous shared language of terms, concepts, and names becomes evident. The language used to describe herbs will have an impact on the way they are perceived and thought about.

We have today a Tower of Babel of plant names. This linguistic richness brings with it both insights and impediments. An example can be seen in the diversity of names for the same plant, or the same name used for different plants, as well as the cornucopia/profusion of regional names, reflective of the rich folklore associated with herbs. This abundant matrix of herb names, which should inform our explorations, is all too often a source of confusion.

Science and Nomenclature Confusion

Binomial nomenclature is a system used in science to name all living beings. Each name is composed of two parts—hence the term *binomial*. The first part of the name identifies the genus to which the organism belongs, while the second part identifies the species within the genus.

A species is the fundamental component of biological classification and is comprised of individuals that share a genetic heritage and can interbreed and produce fertile offspring. A genus is a group of species that are closely related through common descent, with similar traits, qualities, or features. For example, consider the 350 or so species of skullcap; they all belong to the *Scutellaria* genus, but each species has its own specific phylogenetic heritage, regionality, and chemistry.

Although binomial names are known colloquially as the "Latin names," they also make use of several other languages, such as classical Greek, among others. Even in such cases, however, the non-Latin words are latinized.

This is not the place to explore the depth and breadth of taxonomy, but we can note that the value of the binomial system goes way beyond purely scientific utility. The names themselves often offer insights about the plants they are assigned to, whether historical, folkloric, or scientific.

Consider the astounding richness to be found in color names. The botanical lexicography of flower color is as lavish as the abundance it describes. For example, in his classic volume *Botanical Latin*, first published in 1966, British botanist William Stearn listed 103 categories of Latin color terms used as species names, of which 35 are terms for shades of green alone. The English word *green* is completely inadequate to describe the magnificence of the green spectrum on display in an English oak wood. Just two of the many botanical descriptors embedded in plant species names are *viridis*, meaning green, and *glaucus*, sea green. White might be denoted with the prefix *galacto-*, meaning milk white, or with *albidus*, whitish. The glorious yellows of spring might be described as *aureus*, meaning golden yellow, or *luteus*, simply yellow.

Some names highlight visible features, as in St. John's wort, which is characterized by small perforations along the leaf edges, hence its species name *perforatum*. The species name of yarrow is *millefolium*, meaning finely cut, from the Latin *mille* (thousand) and *folium* (leaf).

Names can suggest a strong odor, pleasant or unpleasant. It must be remembered in these days of aromatherapy that not all plants have a sweet bouquet. Disagreeable odors are suggested by such names as *foetidus*, as in *Symplocarpus foetidus* (skunk cabbage). The uniquely lovely bouquet of violet is hinted at in the species name *odorata*, meaning sweet-smelling.

It sometimes seems that every plant name used in classical Greek has been used in modern nomenclature. *Psyllium* comes from the Greek word *psylla*, or flea. Psylla was the Greek name for psyllium, the seeds of which resemble fleas.

A variety of names are taken from classical mythology, often Greek or European, a reflection of the Eurocentric origins of the system (though increasingly binomials are becoming more multicultural). The genus name of yarrow is *Achillea*, from the Greek Achilles, hero of Homer's *Iliad*, whose bleeding ankle was treated with yarrow. The genus *Artemisia* is named for the Greek Artemis, goddess of the hunt. *Angelica archangelica* is said to bloom on the feast day of St. Michael the Archangel, according to the old Julian calendar.

The use of names of people (often naturalists or biologists but also other worthies) is common. The important medicinal genus *Lobelia* is named for Matthias de l'Obel, a Flemish botanist (1538–1616). The genus of the dawn redwood, *Metasequoia*, is named after the Cherokee chief Sequoia, inventor of the Cherokee written language. However, he probably never saw a redwood—these trees do not grow in the region where he lived.

An example of a common name deriving from that of a person is joe-pye weed. Several species carry the name, but it is primarily *Eupatorium purpureum* that is known as joe-pye weed in North American herbalism. There has been much debate about the origin of the name—whether Joe Pye was a real or fictional person, when and where he lived, what his ethnicity was. A 2017 study concluded that Joe Pye was Joseph Shauquethqueat, a Mohican sachem who lived in Massachusetts and New York in the eighteenth and early nineteenth century and is credited with having halted a typhus epidemic in colonial Massachusetts (Pearce 2017, 178, 185).

Pharmaceutical Latin

There is yet another source of technically accurate, "pseudo Latin" names applied to herbs. The names of herbal medicines compounded and dispensed by pharmacists was for many years in a form of Latin that came to be called pharmaceutical Latin. These names are quite accurate within the scholarly specialty but swell the confusing complexity of herb nomenclature.

Pharmakon

Pharmaceutical Latin, an expression of the language of medicine as well as aspects of intellectual life in Europe, goes back a long way. The etymological core of the modern words *pharmacology*, *pharmacy*, and *pharmacopoeia* is much richer than a word meaning simply "drug." The word in question is the ancient Greek *pharmakon*, itself a composite of three meanings: remedy, poison, and scapegoat. In ancient Greek, *pharmakon* can be translated as "drug" but can mean both remedy and poison; it is either the cure of an illness or its cause. The third sense of a scapegoat refers to the *pharmakos* ritual. This was a sacrificial ritual, a kind of societal catharsis, used to shut out evil, out of the body and out of the city. *Pharmakos* was the name given to a human scapegoat who was chosen to become an "outsider" to expiate the city's "ills," being expelled from the community in times of disaster (famine, invasion, or plague) when purification was needed.

Pharmaceutical Latin was once common in official pharmacopoeias. For example, the titles of monographs—descriptions of drugs, including the conditions and limitations for which they may be used, directions for use, warnings, and other information that their labeling must contain—were at one time written in pharmaceutical Latin.

The use of pharmacopoeial Latin in practice was abandoned many years ago. It is considered an obscure corner of the history of pharmacy. However, no matter how modern we consider ourselves as herbalists, referring to historical monographs is unavoidable. With so few people being conversant in Latin of any flavor, the possibility for confusion abounds.

The use of the "Official Latin Title" in monographs was established to ensure precision and accuracy in prescription writing. Latin was chosen as it is not a living language and so was assumed to not change over time. In the nineteenth century, when pharmacopoeial science was developing, Latin was considered the language of science and universally used—today it is not! Monograph titles were latinized, and as such might use the Latin name of the plant, but the rules of Latin grammar took precedence. For example, the important herb belladonna has the Latin name *Atropa belladonna*, but for grammatical reasons monographs would use the name Belladonnae as the title.

With plant medicines, we most commonly see that the pharmaceutical Latin name denotes the geographical region of origin—easily understood, though of little utility. As an example, consider the commonly used Chinese-Western herb differentiation. A pharmaceutical Latin name might indicate that an herb comes from China or, for example, a Western country like Wales, but does this mean it is indigenous to that country or simply cultivated in that country? Does it mean that the herb is a traditional component of that region's system of medicine? How does that affect our understanding of herbs used in more than one regional system of medicine? Consider burdock root, an important remedy in TCM and Western herbalism, but used in different ways and forms, often for different indications. So quite apart from burdock's origins, a pharmaceutical Latin geographical name might have important therapeutic implications.

"Common" Names

Another confusing factor is government attempts at regulation of common names. Government-determined "official common names" are used to facilitate the trade of herbs in the marketplace in order to help consumers identify which herbs they are actually purchasing. As understandable as this goal might be, the absurdities that this shotgun marriage of herbalism and governmental mindset creates can best be seen with the plant the U.S. herbal community knows as Siberian ginseng. Siberian ginseng is not a proper ginseng (that is, it is not in the *Panax* genus), and its binomial was *Eleutherococcus senticosus*, and so to prevent any possible confusion of Siberian ginseng with, say, Asian ginseng (*Panax ginseng*), the government chose *eleuthero* as its new official commercial common name. However, a couple of years after this purely bureaucratic wordplay, taxonomists changed the Latin name of Siberian ginseng to *Acanthopanax senticosus*. The end result of this semantic butchery, meant to help commerce, means that *A. senticosus* is now known as eleuthero, enshrining a name that will make sense only to herbalists and a very few taxonomists!

The commonly used medicinal and culinary herb rosemary has also undergone taxonomic review (de Macedo et al. 2020). It has long been classified as *Rosmarinus officinalis*. However, phylogenetic analysis led to the merging of the genus *Rosmarinus* into the genus *Salvia*. So rosemary could no longer carry the *Rosmarinus* genus name, but it also couldn't simply become *Salvia officinalis* because that name already belongs to culinary sage. So now rosemary is known under the name *Salvia rosmarinus*. This will cause no confusion at all. . . .

In most of the world, the names for common plants can be very variable, reflecting local history and traditions. In the United Kingdom, for example, the name *bachelor's button* has historically been given to about thirty plants. In Somerset, *bachelor's button* is a name for burdock; in the Midlands, it's a double-flowered form of sneezewort; in the West Country, it's feverfew. Tansy (*Tanacetum vulgare*), too, is widely known as bachelor's button, possibly because of its historical use as an abortifacient!

The so-called common name of an herb is often a main source of confusion between plants. To explore this, consider sage and the genus *Salvia*. *Salvia* is one the largest genera of plants, with an estimated seven hundred to nearly a thousand species. The name *Salvia* derives from the Latin *salvere*, meaning "to feel well and healthy," "health," or "heal."

Sage has numerous common names. Some of the best-known include sage, broadleaf sage, common sage, culinary sage, dalmatian sage, garden sage, golden sage, kitchen sage, and true sage. Of course, this is just considering names in English. Every language and geographical region will have their own cornucopia of names rich in history and meaning.

However, *Salvia* is only one of several genera commonly referred to as sage. In addition, consider *Phlomis*, which has several species called sage, including Jerusalem sage (*Phlomis fruticosa*). *Artemisia tridentata* is the common sagebrush, also known as white sage. Next is antelope sage (*Eriogonum jamesii*) and even Texas sage (*Leucophyllum frutescens*).

While *sage* is one name for many plants, the opposite issue can arise too: one plant may carry many names. There is usually a dominant common name for an herb, though sometimes that depends on where the user lives. Consider the well-known plant calendula, which plays an important role in both herbal medicine and natural cosmetics. The binomial is *Calendula officinalis*, and the plant is known as calendula in the United States, but it is called marigold in England.

Historically, marigolds are in the genus *Tagetes* and are native to the Americas. These marigolds were important ceremonial flowers for the Aztecs and so came to the attention of the European colonizers. In the early 1500s, marigolds were among the newly discovered plants sent back to the Old World. The tall *Tagetes erecta* came to England from North Africa and the smaller *T. patula* from France, leading the renowned English herbalist John Gerard to call them African marigold and French marigold in his *Herball or Generall Historie of Plantes*, published in 1599.

Unfortunately, the name *marigold* was already in use in England when these plants arrived. The plant usually called a marigold was the yellow/orange flower named *Calendula officinalis*. There were other marigolds in England, all with yellow/orange flowers, like marsh marigold and corn marigold. But the calendula was the one most people called a marigold.

Upon arriving in England, the new marigolds grew easily and became very popular. As they eclipsed the earlier marigold (*Calendula*), people started calling the *Tagetes* species simply marigolds, and the *Calendula* species had to be called pot marigold in order not to confuse them.

Chemical and Drug Names

When a drug is first discovered, it is given a chemically specific name describing its molecular structure. Chemical names are usually too complex and awkward for general use, so either a shorthand version of the name or a code name (such as RU 486) is developed for ease of use. When a chemical studied for pharmacological use is approved for human or veterinary use, it is given both a generic and a brand name. The generic name is assigned by an official body—in the United States, it is the United States Adopted Names (USAN) Council. The brand name is developed by the company requesting approval for the drug and identifies it as the exclusive property of that company.

The potential for confusion is well illustrated with the herbal history and naming of aspirin. A ubiquitous drug, aspirin is a mild analgesic useful in the relief of headache and muscle and joint aches. It works by inhibiting the production of prostaglandins, chemicals produced by the body with a range of functions. They are necessary for blood clotting but also sensitize nerve endings to pain.

To be chemically specific, aspirin is acetylsalicylic acid, a derivative of salicylic acid, which in turn is derived from willow, of the genus *Salix*. Willow's pain-relieving properties have long been known; Hippocrates (460–375 BCE) was familiar with them, and thus willow's use for pain relief must have predated classical Greece.

In the early nineteenth century, scientists discovered that a compound called salicin, found in the bark of willows, was pain relieving. In the body, salicin is converted to salicylic acid. This led pharmacologists

to the development of salicylic acid, which is an effective and mild analgesic, but unfortunately it causes stomach inflammation. Mixing the
salicylic acid with acetyl chloride neutralized the acidity and produced
acetylsalicylic acid. It was commercialized under the trademarked name
Aspirin and patented on February 27, 1900. The name *Aspirin* comes
from the initial *A* in *acetyl chloride*, the *spir* in *Spiraea* (the former genus
name for meadowsweet, the plant from which pharmacologists derived
the salicylic acid; today it is known as *Filipendula ulmaria*), and the use
of *in* as a then-familiar name ending for medicines. Thus, the chemical
name is derived from the name of willow, and the commonly used commercial name (which started as the proprietary name) is derived from
the name of meadowsweet.

For most people in the twenty-first century's dominant culture, herbalism is outside the realm of their daily lives, and some might consider it
fringe or even exotic. It is, however, a core component of human life—
in fact, it is a birthright for being part of the biosphere on planet Earth.
An exploration of herbalism, seeing its presence in and contributions to
culture, suggests the need for a map to facilitate the journey. However,
maps are nothing more than scale models of reality, symbolically depict-
ing relationships between things, such as geographic features. They are
symbols, not the reality itself. For maps to be useful, their symbology
needs to be understood. Mistaking the map for the territory is a logical fallacy that occurs when someone confuses the semantics of a term
with what the term represents. So as much as there needs to be an
understanding of the language used to describe herbalism's map, this
language is not herbalism.

The only conclusion to all this potential confusion is to recognize
that context is everything here. The language of herbalism seems to
vary with the milieu in which it is being discussed. This is not a minor
quibble but rather is indicative of the need to build bridges between
worldviews in the wide world of herbalism today—between science-
based phytotherapy and folk herbalism, regulators of herbal products,
and the people consuming them.

PART TWO

The Science

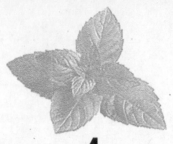

4

An Old Herbalist Looks at the New Science

Using herbalism and the human experience of herbs as a lens, the world is revealed as a synergistic, integrated whole that is to be celebrated for its diversity. *Synergy* refers to cooperative effects produced by things that interact or work together. Although it is often defined as "the whole being more than the sum of its parts," it is much more than that, as cooperation can take many forms, from simple additive effects to complex emergent phenomena. Cooperative interactions are everywhere in nature, but the recognition of synergy shifts the focus from mechanistic explanations to the relationships among things, and the effects these relationships produce. Synergy is a ubiquitous and fundamental aspect of the natural world. As such, it is also fundamental to herbalism, though it is still a controversial concept in medicine and pharmacology, where the "one disease–one target–one drug" mindset still reigns.

On the heels of the Human Genome Project and its cornucopia of new science, new technologies have revolutionized the perspective, tools, and insights through which herbalism can be seen. Plants and the insights derived from the practice of herbal medicine have much to offer modern health care, well beyond the search for superdrugs. The mainstream is recognizing that support of homeostasis, integration, and resilience are areas of meaningful research. The use of herbs easily fits into both the perspectives of the new science and the array of new protocols being developed. And though clinicians may not always realize it, science and medicine are now using principles that assume complex synergistic interactions.

The newly developed "omics" technologies adopt a holistic view of the molecules that make up an organism, with the ultimate aim being to understand the complexity of whole systems. The key insight is that a complex system can be understood more thoroughly if it is considered as a whole, and evolving technology has created tools that enable this. As an example, consider metabolomics.

Metabolomics studies chemical processes involving metabolites, measuring broad changes caused by specific stimuli and identifying the fingerprint of biochemical changes within cells. Such a comprehensive evaluation of the metabolic state helps identify changes that are characteristic of both disease states and health. This means that a comprehensive description of molecular functioning in life processes has become a real possibility (Yan et al. 2015).

Metabolomics is becoming a valuable tool in recognizing compounds connected with activity in herbal medicines. Cellular alterations caused by even highly complex herbal mixtures can be measured. The multitude of compounds present may act on specific targets, but the observed biological activity is the result of combined effects. This holistic/synergist view is held by most of the world's herb traditions. However, recognition of the multitarget actions of the many constituents present in any formulation has been a profound challenge for phytotherapeutic research (Liu et al. 2012).

Herbal medicine has much to expect from the cornucopia of data flowing from the new technologies, rich as it is in insights derived through the integration of perspectives of systems biology and network pharmacology. Systems biology is a holistic approach to understanding the complexity of biological systems. It studies the interactions and behavior of the components of biological systems such as molecules, cells, organs, and organisms. It is predicated on the insight that networks forming the whole of living organisms cannot be explained by studying their components, as the system is more than the sum of its parts. This leads to the idea of biology as a network of networks. From genomes to molecules to cells to organs to body systems to organisms in their world, biology is fundamentally a network of networks.

Network Pharmacology

Network pharmacology applies holistic principles to pharmacology, seeking to understand how substances (herb, drug, or food) affect the body as a single complex biological system. Instead of considering the effect of a drug to be the result of one specific drug-protein interaction, it sees the outcome of the network of interactions a drug may have. Network pharmacology embraces the complexities of life.

Herbal medicine has become a rich field for such research, especially the exploration of synergistic interactions of two or more herbs. Technologies that allow us to compare gene activity induced by herbal extracts has made it possible to study such synergistic interactions in the human body. The fundamentally holistic perspective of network pharmacology encourages a shift in focus from single-target single-drug therapies to network-targeted multicomponent therapeutics.

The term *network target* refers to the categorization of a disease-specific biomolecular network as a therapeutic target. Researchers have realized that the disruption of biomolecular networks can act as sensors and drivers of common human diseases. The mechanism of action of an herbal formula might be to adjust some component of pharmacological activity, not for single molecules, but for imbalances in the status of these disease-specific networks.

The world being revealed by all these new technologies seems to grow ever more complex. Instead of illuminating the underlying "laws" of the physical world (as science once thought it would), they unveil a reality of profound complexity and interrelatedness, with a growing appreciation of the relationships between (and within) wholes and parts and between various levels of organization. In the 1960s, science promised to offer us "better living through chemistry;" today, we might say that it offers "better living through ecology!"

Primary and Secondary Metabolites

Metabolites are organic compounds synthesized by both plants and animals via metabolic pathways. In other words, they are the intermediate or end products of metabolism, the total sum of chemical reactions that take place within the cells of an organism to produce energy. The plant kingdom as a whole is estimated to produce between two hundred thousand and one million metabolites, with any given species thought to contain upward of five thousand metabolites.

Plant metabolites are of two types: primary and secondary. Primary metabolites are indispensable to life processes and so are found universally among all plants. Examples are energy-rich fuel molecules, such as sucrose and starch, as well as DNA, RNA, and pigments such as chlorophyll.

Secondary metabolites have little to do with the inner life of a plant's cell but are deeply involved in the individual organism's interactions with its environment. These chemicals tend to be unique, have a widely diverse array of structures, and are adaptive for the plant and/or species. Without these compounds, many key physiological processes would cease, with catastrophic consequences on ecosystem functionality.

New technologies and their application by the omics sciences are revealing a world of interactions, of chemical relationships, that herbal secondary metabolites are perfectly suited to. Some secondary metabolites—often those most familiar to Western medicine—appear to be specific for one or a limited number of molecular targets. These are the few but dramatic plant constituents that most closely approximate the classic definition of a "drug," such as the alkaloids scopolamine and the cardiac glycoside digoxin. However, most plants used in herbal medicine do not contain markedly active compounds and usually are used in the form of an extract that might contain hundreds of metabolites. In most cases, it is almost impossible to define a single chemical that explains the bioactivity of the extract; instead, its activity is likely due to the synergistic interactions of many of the metabolites, and that synergism cannot be detected when single compounds are evaluated alone.

The basis for any pharmacological understanding of herb activity is the pleiotropic characteristics of the herb's metabolites—that is, their dynamic interactions with multiple targets (Wink 2008). Such multi-target effects take many forms but appear to be facilitated by some basic processes. As an example, one fundamental metabolite-driven process is modulation of macromolecules, which affects the activity of proteins, which in turn may affect the whole gamut of cellular organelles and activity. Plant metabolites have been shown to modulate cellular receptors, enzymes, ion channels, ion pumps, elements of the cytoskeleton, membranes, and much more. The ability to modulate the three-dimensional structure of proteins, and so their function, appears to be universal. Additionally, herbal complexes may contain synergists that can interact with cytochrome P450 enzymes or enhance the absorption and thus bioavailability of active metabolites (Dixon et al. 2007).

The Paradigm Shift

A revolution in perspectives, tools, and insights has occurred in biology. This is not an exaggeration, it is simply an observation, and it may best be described as a paradigm shift—not theoretical or idealized, but actually a paradigm shift. That phrase, *paradigm shift*, originated in a 1962 book titled *The Structure of Scientific Revolutions*, which transformed the philosophy of science and the way scientists think about their work. Its author, Thomas Kuhn, saw scientific endeavor as being characterized by two quite different types of change. The first was the kind of incremental change that typifies the daily course of "normal" science. The second was the kind of revolutionary change that disrupts normality. This sort of scientific revolution does not result from the slow, steady advance of knowledge but involves a paradigm shift—a fundamental change in basic concepts and practices, in marked contrast to science done within a prevailing framework (or paradigm). The paradigm is not simply the current theory but the entire worldview in which that theory exists, and all of the implications that come with it.

The holistic perspectives of systems biology and network pharmacology being explored in this new paradigm are proving to be key for our investigation of herbalism and the potential role of medicinal plants in modern holistic medicine. Why are these modern sciences so relevant to the ancient art and science of herbalism? What follows is a very brief overview of some of the more relevant aspects that will inform the rest of the book.

The "Omics" Revolution

The genome is the total DNA of an organism, and genomics is the study of all the genes in an organism. Genomics involves sequencing DNA as well as identifying the function of the encoded genes. It was once thought that sequencing the human genome would immediately tell us the identity of human genes. However, the genome has proved to be much more multifaceted and complex!

The rapidly evolving technology that originated with the Human Genome Project has led to research tools that enable a more holistic study of biological systems. Experimental techniques have been developed that increase throughput, such as microarrays, enabling evaluation of the changes in many genes or proteins simultaneously. Such high-throughput screening enables thousands of tests to be conducted at the same time, allowing the simultaneous study of the expression and activity of thousands of genes, metabolites, and proteins. By allowing the characterization and quantification of large collections of biological molecules at once, it offers a potential window into the life and dynamics of an organism. With this technology, the challenge is not to generate data but to interpret it (Rai, Saito, and Yamazaki 2017).

The English-language neologism *omics* informally refers to a field of study in biology, such as genomics or metabolomics, dedicated to the quantitative analysis of a complete or near-complete assortment of all the constituents of a system. Omics technologies provide the tools needed to interpret the sort of massive data collections gathered by high-throughput genomic screening. The key omics insight is that a complex system can be understood more thoroughly if considered as a whole. Metabolomics is especially relevant to herbalism and is explored below, but there are many areas of omics studies, including genomics (genes), transcriptomics (transcripts or messenger RNA), and proteomics (proteins).

Metabolomics

Omics is leading to some dramatic developments in our understanding of metabolite activity. As noted earlier, secondary metabolites have a unique and vast chemical diversity and, through the natural selection process, have evolved for optimal interactions with biological macromolecules (Hong 2011). The term *metabolome* encapsulates the total collection of metabolites in a cell, tissue, or organism at a given point in time and under specific physiological conditions (Shafi and Zahoor 2021). It is a snapshot of an organism's in-the-moment biochemistry. The very ambitious goal of metabolomics is to qualitatively and quantitatively analyze all the metabolites in an organism in order to identify and measure changes in the metabolome. Such a comprehensive evaluation of the metabolic state can help us identify changes that are characteristic of specific disease states—that is, the fingerprint of biochemical changes that indicate imbalances.

For traditional herbal medicines, metabolomics is also a major tool for identifying active constituents. Before the onset of omics technologies, screening tests focused on the activity of individual compounds at the molecular level in, for example, receptor binding assays. This is not the best approach for studies on traditional medicines because it doesn't account for synergistic interactions and dynamic cascades of effects. A more holistic approach using systems biology seems better suited to prove the efficacy of herbal remedies and obtain information that might lead to understanding their mode of action. Synergy, prodrugs, novel targets—all these might be detected by a systems biology approach, whereas the reductionist approach will recognize only activity on already known targets.

How Many Metabolites Are Involved?

In the understated language of science, measuring the immense number of plant metabolites is "nontrivial"! It is estimated that there are approximately four hundred thousand species of vascular plants on Earth, which are the source of hundreds of thousands of metabolites (Willis 2017).

Plant primary metabolism is substantially similar to that of non-plants. However, plants and fungi have additional capacity to synthesize an enormous repertoire of specialized (or secondary) compounds. In fact, plants display far greater metabolic diversity than other organisms. As discussed later, the vast majority of plant metabolites are variations on a theme resulting from one or more structural modifications of a common (carbon) backbone. Common examples are nitrogen-containing compounds, phenolics, flavonoids, and terpenes.

The plant kingdom is thought to contain between two hundred thousand and one million metabolites, with any given species containing upward of five thousand metabolites. Secondary metabolites account for the majority of this diversity (Dixon and Strack 2003).

Pleiotropy

Until recently, the search for new pharmaceutical drugs was characterized by the "one disease–one target–one drug" approach. Its primacy in research is not because of adherence to the central dogma but to facilitate and streamline screening tests for particular compounds and simplify the registration process. But this approach oversimplifies disease mechanisms, which are in fact complex networks of biochemical interactions (Casas et al. 2019).

In revealing the multifaceted pharmacology underlying everything, metabolomics highlights the need for medicines that do a range of relevant things at once. For this, we turn to *pleiotropy*. The term derives from the Greek *pleio*, "many," and *tropic*, "affecting." In genetics, *pleiotropy* describes a single gene that controls multiple phenotypic traits. In pharmacology, it describes all of a drug's actions other than those for which it was specifically developed. In herbalism, it describes the terrain-specific multitargeted effects of plant compounds.

Metabolomics is showing us that many secondary metabolites are pleiotropic, having the potential of simultaneously inhibiting and modulating several factors. As an example, we can consider quercetin, named after *Quercus*, the oak genus. Quercetin is one of the most abundant flavonoids in many medicinal plants and in the human diet, and it has been shown to have pleiotropic effects. To begin, its antitumor activity has been repeatedly confirmed. Quercetin appears to impact multiple intracellular targets, affecting different cell signaling processes in cancer cells. Simultaneously targeting multiple pathways may help kill malignant cells and slow the development of drug resistance.

Its molecular structure endows quercetin with strong antioxidant and anti-inflammatory activities, which makes it beneficial for cardiovascular diseases, such as hypertension. It exerts antiallergy effects by inhibiting the release of histamine from mast cells. It can significantly promote cell apoptosis and inhibit blood vessel generation and transfer. It also has antibacterial activity and effectively reduces the formation of biofilms (Russo, Russo, and Spagnuolo 2014).

Quercetin and other flavonoids exert multiple beneficial effects on the vascular system, including cerebrovascular blood flow, and have the potential to protect neurons against neurotoxins. They are currently being investigated for their use in preventing age-related neurodegeneration (Vauzour et al. 2008).

Herbal Insights That Flow from Omics

The array of omics technology has the potential to transform our understanding of herbs with powerful analytical tools comprehensively profiling secondary metabolites and their actual pharmacology. This is facilitating insights about mode of action, bioavailability, and pharmacokinetics. It also facilitates the observation and assessment of the safety of herbal medicines.

To begin, evaluation of the purity of herbal medicines is essential in their quality control. Current methods used for quality control are based on the detection of chemical markers of constituents. Using metabolomics, the standardized metabolic fingerprint of an herbal product can be generated. Such metabolomics-based fingerprinting aids in the identification of adulteration that is crucial for patient safety.

Metabolomics also allows us to measure changes in cellular biochemistry caused by highly complex herb mixtures. The multitude of compounds present may act on specific targets, but the biological activity is the result of combined effects.

Gene expression profiling is, like metabolomics, an omics technique; it identifies which genes are active in a cell at any given moment, measuring thousands of genes at a time. In one study, gene expression profiling in human nerve cells was examined with and without treatment by an herb mixture consisting of eleuthero root, schisandra berry, and rhodiola root (Panossian et al. 2007). The secondary metabolites of these herbs are well known and include eleutheroside E, schizandrin B, and salidroside. The study found that this combination of phytochemicals activated specific genes that were found not to be affected by the single compounds, suggesting synergistic interactions in the mixture. In other words, omics proves that the chemical whole is more than simply the sum of its chemical parts (Panossian et al. 2013).

The synergy unveiled by the above study is part of what makes evaluating the pharmacological activity of medicinal plants so challenging. With metabolomics, however, we can profile the metabolites in the entire organism that alter in responses to illness, identify their related metabolic pathways, and clarify the mechanism of drug or herb actions. For example, metabolomic research into the mechanisms and impact of traditional herbal formulations on the health of the liver is well established in China (Xiong 2018). Acute liver failure is a life-threatening disorder that has been treated successfully with the traditional Chinese medicine formulation known as Ma Huang Decoction (MHD). First described in the third-century Treatise on Febrile Disease, it contains ma huang, bitter apricot kernel, and licorice, and it has traditionally been used in treating asthma, coughs, and colds. In a study to clarify the mechanisms of MHD in treating acute liver failure, researchers identified thirty-six metabolites contributing to liver failure and found that MHD normalized perturbations in twenty-seven of them (Liao et al. 2021). Interpreting the protective effect against acute liver failure, the researchers found that MHD works mainly through regulation of the Krebs cycle and amino acid metabolism.

The richness of pharmacological interactions shown by herbs and their constituents points to their potential diversity of roles in physiology and thus health and wholeness. This subtle yet profound involvement is not unique to our species but indicative of an ecological role in environmental health and wholeness. Because the physiology of homeostasis is fundamental at all levels of biology, a role for secondary metabolites in the ecology of the biosphere should come as no surprise.

5

The Ecological Theater and the Evolutionary Play

S ynergy is integral to evolution because cooperating organisms gain survival advantage. The term *synergy* comes from Greek *sun*, "together," and *ergon*, "work," and is generally taken to mean two or more things working together to create a combined effect that is greater than the effect of each in isolation. The concept of synergy is fundamental to herbalism, and that idea, supported by an abundance of examples of herbs and their secondary metabolites, fills the rest of the book.

Synergy is one possible—and common—outcome of symbiosis. The word *symbiosis* comes from the Greek *sym*, "together," and *bios*, "life," and denotes two or more organisms living together in intimate relationship. The importance of symbiosis to all life on Earth cannot be overstated. In every ecological community, symbiotic relationships are crucial to maintaining balance in nature's multiple processes. They can take many forms, one being a mutualistic relationship between two species that support each other by doing things for each other that they can't do alone. Symbiosis played a major role in the coevolution of flowering plants and the animals that pollinate them. Plants get pollinated, and pollinators receive a range of benefits, depending on the species. Most pollinators are nurtured by pollen or nectar, but some bees, for example, also use wax and resin from flowers to build their hives. In one especially unique mutualism, male orchid bees collect fragrant pollen from various orchid flowers and turn the aromatic oils into sex pheromones—that is, "perfume" to attract mates. A male bee uses his forelegs to collect the pollen for storage on his hind legs, and in the process, the pollen gets onto the bee's back, where it can rub off and pollinate other flowers.

Symbiosis not only contributes to evolution but actually may be central as *the* source of evolutionary innovation through a process called *symbiogenesis*, which translates as "becoming by living together." It seems that symbiosis facilitates much evolutionary innovation, with modern animal and plant cells resulting from endosymbiosis, a symbiotic partnership in which one species lives *inside the cells* of another (Wiser 2022). Mitochondria and chloroplasts are the two most widespread, ancient, and ecologically important endosymbioses. Mitochondria were once free-living bacteria that took up residence inside the cells of our unicellular ancestors well over a billion years ago. They are now a critical part of cellular machinery, acting as the "power plants" of cells. All the multicellular organisms—fungi, plants, animals—have mitochondria descended from that first engulfed bacterium. Similarly, chloroplasts—the structures within plant cells that photosynthesize—descend from an endosymbiosis with cyanobacteria (Margulis and Sagan 2002).

This integrative ecology, and its patterns of synergy, can be seen at every level of organization, whether it be the chemistry of the plant, relationships with pollinators and herbivores, or the pharmacology of herbal medicine. In the natural world, synergistic phenomena are ubiquitous. Synergy has been suggested as a factor that can explain the progressive evolution of complexity in living systems, with synergistic effects underlying cooperative relationships of all kinds and at all levels in living systems.

A basic principle in ecology is the fundamental importance of diversity, because the more diverse an ecosystem is, the more stable it is. When we talk about ecological diversity, most often we mean biodiversity. As the American Museum of Natural History's Center for

Biodiversity and Conservation sums it up: "The term biodiversity (from 'biological diversity') refers to the variety of life on Earth at all its levels, from genes to ecosystems, and can encompass the evolutionary, ecological, and cultural processes that sustain life" (American Museum of Natural History, n.d.).

Biodiversity plays a central mythic and symbolic role in our language, religion, literature, art, and music, making it a key component of human culture with benefits to society that have not been quantified but are clearly vast. Humans have never lived in a world with low biodiversity. We've always been dependent on a varied and rich natural environment for both our physical survival and our psychological and spiritual health.

Underpinning that great diversity of life is a matrix of profound *chemodiversity*. As omics technologies are beginning to show us, we live in an ocean of chemical interactions, a vast ecology of chemistry, and chemodiversity is just as crucial to and reflective of life on Earth as biodiversity.

Plant secondary metabolites are often facilitators of symbiotic interfaces. In terms of the plant-human relationship, every medicinal herb contains several constituents underlying its therapeutic-to-humans properties. The abundance of metabolite diversity and remarkable range of properties raises the question: Why? What role do these metabolites play in the plant, in the environment, and in people? Exploration of their ecological role illustrates the deep and intense coevolutionary relationships that characterize life on Earth.

The Ecological Role
of Secondary Metabolites

The range of ecological roles played by the diversity of secondary metabolites is truly impressive. An insight to take from this is that secondary metabolites are physiologically important compounds originating from adaptation processes driven by natural selection. In other words, the vast majority of secondary metabolites can be assumed to fulfill a physiological function that would bring a selective advantage (Jenke-Kodama, Müller, and Dittmann 2008). They are important modifiers of biodiversity, influencing the ecology of plant communities in constantly changing environments. Secondary metabolites increase a plant's overall ability to survive and overcome local challenges by allowing it to interact with its environment (Harborne 1993). In fact, they play pivotal roles as communication signals in complex ecological communities. Even a cursory look at the ecological role of secondary metabolites reveals a multitude of examples.

Defense

Chemical warfare as a relevant metaphor became influential in the 1960s, when secondary metabolites were interpreted as fulfilling a purely defensive/aggressive role, acting as an arsenal for "natural" chemical warfare. Many secondary metabolites undoubtedly act as effective defensive weapons, but from a more nuanced ecological perspective, this defensive posture is only part of the complex matrix of interactions the plant is involved with.

Secondary metabolites play a fundamental role in plants' defense against microorganisms, such as bacteria, fungi, and viruses, as well as herbivores. They can be protective in other ways, such as being antioxidant, ultraviolet-light-absorbing, and antiproliferative agents. Most significantly, they also manage interplant relationships, defending a plant's growing space against competitor plants.

Secondary metabolites from plants may be used by insects for defense. For example, some insects store these plant metabolites in their bodies. The metabolites influence the growth, survival, and reproduction of these insects and other organisms, whether beneficially or detrimentally.

Attraction

Of equal importance is the role of secondary metabolites in plants' symbiotic relationships. Consider a plant's attraction of pollinators and other symbiotes via color or scent or the provision of indirect defense for the plant by attracting the natural enemies of its herbivorous attackers. The latter may take the form of providing an attractive chemical milieu for the predator or, alternatively, may be in direct response to tissue damage by the herbivore, which results in the synthesis and release of a cocktail of phytochemicals that attract the herbivore's natural predators.

Recognition

Most insects feed or lay eggs on a limited number of plants, often those species belonging to a single plant family. In many cases, their ability to find the appropriate plants lies in their recognition of a unique combination of secondary metabolites, which they detect using a range of senses, including sight, smell, taste, and touch. For some species, such as butterflies whose larvae eat only one particular plant species, recognition of the chemical signature of the plant's secondary metabolites is crucial.

Insect Sex

Insects produce pheromones to attract the opposite sex. These compounds are strictly species-specific, with unique chemical structures and/or combinations of components manufactured by specific biosynthetic pathways. However, in some instances, insects employ certain secondary metabolites from plants to attract and excite the partners during courtship.

Males of the danaine butterfly species *Idea leuconoe* have what are known as hair pencils, brush-like glandular organs used to excrete pheromones that act as aphrodisiacs and tranquilizers to females as well as repellents to other males. Some of the pheromone compounds that are produced in hair pencils, such as pyrrolizidine alkaloids, come from plants (Nishida 2014).

Types of Secondary Metabolites

Secondary metabolites can be categorized into a number of distinct groups based on their chemical structure. The main groups are the alkaloids, phenolic compounds, and terpenes. Terpenes are particularly important to our subject, and so they are the focus of much of the following discussion.

Alkaloids

Alkaloids are a group of more than three thousand nitrogen-containing compounds that are found in more than 20 percent of plant species. They are often distinguished on the basis of a structural similarity. While not all alkaloids have a major impact on the body, the diverse array of pharmacological actions demonstrated by various alkaloids includes analgesia, local anesthesia, cardiac stimulation, respiratory stimulation and relaxation, vasoconstriction, muscle relaxation, and toxicity, as well as antineoplastic, hypertensive, and hypotensive properties.

Alkaloids can pose major cultural issues because of their properties. They provide humanity with challenges, such as nicotine, heroin, and cocaine, as well as the profound gift of visionary entheogens, such as psilocybin and mescaline. Some alkaloids, such as coniine and strychnine, are extremely toxic, while others, including atropine, codeine, morphine, and vincristine, are used as pharmaceuticals. In terms of their ecological roles, alkaloids primarily act in plants as feeding deterrents and toxins to herbivores.

Phenolics

Phenolics occur ubiquitously in plants, with well over ten thousand known. Being so common in plants, phenolics are an important part of the human diet. Structurally, they share at least one aromatic hydrocarbon ring with one or more hydroxyl groups attached. The simplest compound with this structural motif is phenol, hence the name of the group, and it is modifications of the basic skeleton that produces flavones, flavonols, flavanones, isoflavones, and anthocyanins. Phenolics range from simple compounds, such as the coumarins, to more complex structures, such as flavonoids and tannins. Of these, the flavonoids comprise some six thousand compounds.

Phenolics contribute to a benign palette of intra- and interplant protective, symbiotic, and attractant/deterrent effects. For instance, they are induced in the face of bacterial or fungal attack; they provide scent, color, and flavor to attract symbiotic insects and deter herbivores; they act as phagostimulants; and they manage plants' symbiotic relationships with soil bacteria. Many phenolic compounds also play roles in antioxidant defenses and the absorption of ultraviolet (UV) light.

Flavonoids

Although increasing attention is being given to the role and use of flavonoids in medicine and the food industry, their relevance for plants and the wider ecosystem cannot be overstated. Flavonoids are deeply involved in all aspects of plant life, especially their ecological lives. However, they have a similar range of metabolic effects on the internal life of both plants and animals. They are renowned for their antioxidant properties, but they have much more extensive biological activities. A partial list of pharmacological activities discovered so far shows that flavonoids can be anti-inflammatory, antibacterial, antiviral, antiallergenic, antithrombotic, antiatherosclerotic, vasodilating, hepatoprotective, and antitumor. In particular, this group of molecules appears to have a unique capacity to modulate key cellular enzyme functions.

Of unique relevance to plants is the protection flavonoids offer against damage caused by UV light, which, to some extent, results from the fact that they can act as a sunscreen, absorbing UV radiation and, as they are mainly in the leaves and stems, reducing the penetration of UV light to more vulnerable tissues.

Flavonoids are also released by plant roots and act as specific messengers in symbiotic relations between species. For example, readily available nitrogen in the soil is essential for healthy plant growth, and low nitrogen levels dramatically inhibit plant growth. When soil nitrogen levels are low, some plants respond by producing more flavonoids and so cause a buildup of these molecules in the soil. This, in turn, attracts microbes (called diazotrophs) that fix atmospheric nitrogen gas in the soil in forms available to plants. Flavonoids are also important in the formation of mycorrhiza, the mutually beneficial symbiotic association in which soil-borne fungi colonize the cortical tissues of plant roots (Abdel-Lateif, Bogusz, and Hocher 2012).

Plant-plant interactions can be positive or negative and may depend on the concentrations of flavonoids. The negative relations are mainly based on inhibiting the germination and growth of other plants' seedlings. The flavonoid germination deterrents are usually excreted through roots into the soil but can be also found in leaves and even in pollen, which, after falling onto the surrounding soil, inhibits the germination of other plants.

Flavonoids play a pivotal role in plant resistance against bacteria and fungi. Such properties can be nonspecific and often result from their antioxidative properties. They quench the damaging reactive oxygen ions that are generated both by the pathogens and by the plant as a result of the infection.

Flavonoids are also often pivotal in the relations between plants and animals. They provide color, fragrance, and taste to fruits, flowers, and seeds, making them attractive for insects, birds, or mammals, which aid in pollen or seed transmission. Flavonoids are crucial to the regulation of egg laying for some insects. For example, naringenin, along with other active compounds, stimulates egg laying by the swallowtail butterfly on young leaves of citrus plants (Honda 1990).

As compounds originating in plants, flavonoids are part of the human diet and have many positive impacts on human health—so much so that they are now common components in a variety of nutraceutical, pharmaceutical, medicinal, and cosmetic products. Many flavonoids express antibacterial, antifungal, or antiviral properties. For instance, the common flavonoids apigenin and amentoflavone show strong effects against pathogenic fungi, including *Candida albicans*. As well, the flavonoid kaempferol shows activity against Gram-positive and Gram-negative bacteria, as well as against the fungus *Candida glabrata* (Aboulghazi et al. 2022).

Terpenes

About 60 percent of all secondary metabolites are terpenoids, and more than fifty thousand have been identified (Ninkuu et al. 2021). The etymology of the name *terpene* highlights the human interaction with these constituents. The word originates (via French and Latin) from *turpentine*, which originally described the thick, pleasantly aromatic balsam that flows from the bark of some pines. The Latin root is *ter(e) binthina*, "(resin) of the terebinth tree." The aroma of that resin is the result of its terpenes.

The classical source of turpentine was the terebinth, a Mediterranean tree related to the pistachio. However, various species of pines are used as sources today. The sticky, viscous material exuded by the trees consists of resins (actually oleoresins) dissolved in a volatile oil, which can be distilled. This separates the volatile oil of turpentine from the nonvolatile rosin.

Terpenes are widely found in plants and are familiar as the characteristic aroma molecules of essential oils. The number and diversity of terpenes found in nature is a good indication of how important they are in plant evolution and ecology, which in turn suggests the diversity of pharmacological effects they possess. Among many other qualities, terpenes have the potential to serve as anticancer and antidiabetic medicines, as well as being memory-enhancing acetyl cholinesterase inhibitors that can contribute to the treatment of dementia (Gershenzon and Dudareva 2007).

In terms of toxicity, terpenes range from deadly to entirely benign, reflecting their broad range of ecological roles. In plants, terpenes play a role in everything from attracting insects or birds for the purposes of pollination and seed dispersal to repelling herbivores by being overtly toxic. Other roles include the generation of volatile chemical signals that, in turn, generate aromas and flavors.

Although the structure (and hence activity) of this wonderfully diverse group of secondary metabolites is relatively straightforward, the way they are named can be extremely confusing! Terpenes are constructed of repeated isoprene units and are classified according to the number of isoprene units they contain (see the table below). Isoprene itself is volatile and is released from leaves as a natural by-product of plant metabolism. It is one of the most common organic compounds found in the atmosphere.

CLASSIFICATION OF TERPENES

Classification	Isoprene Units	Carbon Atoms
Monoterpene	2	10
Sesquiterpene	3	15
Diterpene	4	20
Triterpene	6	30

Monoterpenes are abundant; the monoterpene α-pinene has been detected in nearly every green plant. They are small, volatile, active molecules that are characterized by their aromas. Their ecological functions include being signal molecules in the aroma of flowers to attract pollinators. They are also active as defensive molecules, with direct roles against herbivores and plant pathogens and indirect defense signaling to attract natural enemies of herbivores.

Sesquiterpenes, and specifically sesquiterpene lactones, discussed beginning on page 87, may play a significant role in human health, both as part of a balanced diet and as medicine, whether herbal or pharmaceutical.

Diterpenes are found in many plants, animals, and fungi. They form the basis for biologically important compounds such as retinol, retinal, and phytol and have key roles in plant development, defense, and ecological adaptation. Naturally occurring diterpenes exert several biological activities, such as anti-inflammatory, antimicrobial, and antispasmodic properties.

Triterpenes are also a big, widely distributed group. Animals, plants, and fungi all produce triterpenes, including squalene, the precursor to all steroids. Saponins are an important subgroup of triterpenes of great importance in herbal medicine, having an impressive range of pharmacological uses, including being antidiabetic, antifungal, antitumor, antiviral, antiparasitic, anti-inflammatory, and immunomodulatory, as well as facilitating the synthesis of hormones and acting on the cardiovascular system, the central nervous system, and the endocrine system. Some have adaptogenic or hepatoprotective activity. They also decrease blood cholesterol levels and may be used as adjuvants in vaccines. In addition, saponins are used in preparation of soaps, detergents, fire extinguishers, shampoos, beer, and cosmetics. The pharmaceutical industry depends on plant saponins as raw material for the synthesis of steroidal drugs such as birth control medication (Barbosa 2014).

Terpenes are pivotal in the complex of allelopathic interactions between plants in an ecosystem. The term *allelopathy* comes from the Greek *allele*, "one another" or "mutual," and *pathy*, "suffering," and refers to the manner in which some plants use chemical signals to inhibit other plants. It is a survival mechanism that allows a plant to compete with nearby plants by inhibiting seed sprouting, root development, or nutrient uptake.

In mutualistic symbiotic relationships, terpenes play critical roles by serving as messengers among species. Terpenes are good conveyors of information over distances because they are volatile at ordinary temperatures. In addition, the vast structural variety of terpenes present allows messages to be very specific. For example, terpenes make up the messages sent from plants to insects, often acting as pheromones: alarm pheromones, trail pheromones, sex pheromones, and many others. Consider the terpene β-farnesene, which is an alarm pheromone in aphids. To humans, it has a characteristic "green apple" aroma. Released by a plant in response to being eaten, it causes aphids to stop feeding, disperse, and give birth to winged (rather than wingless) forms, which fly away.

The Function of Mixtures

A unique characteristic of terpenes is that they usually occur in complex mixtures that fulfill multiple, differing, or additive ecological roles for the plant. In many cases, these mixtures have been found to work synergistically. Inhibition of the growth of competitor plants appears to work this way, as does insect deterrence. For plants with a wide range of enemies, a diverse combination of terpenes may help achieve simultaneous protection against numerous predators, parasites, and competitors.

The mixture's complexity makes it challenging for insects to evolve resistance.

Terpenes are one of the major components of fruit and flower volatiles. A single flower can emanate more than a hundred terpenoid scent compounds. A plant's diversity of aroma compounds (terpenes) and flower color compounds (flavonoids) will preferentially attract certain insects, such as beetles and butterflies.

Songbirds have been seen adding fresh aromatic plants such as lavender to their nest. Warmth from the nestlings increases release of the terpene-rich essential oil from the plants, thereby reducing bacterial growth in the nest and deterring parasites. The human striving to participate in this terpene experience has been a driving force in the development of, among other pursuits, herbal medicines, perfumes, foods, and cocktails.

Forest Bathing in Terpenes

In 1982, the Japanese Ministry of Agriculture, Forestry, and Fisheries coined the term *shinrin-yoku*, "forest bathing" or "absorbing the forest atmosphere." They were actively encouraging people to spend time in nature, not bathing! The goal of *shinrin-yoku* is to help people practice mindfulness, to live in the present moment, to immerse the senses in the natural setting. Indeed, like mindfulness practices in general, forest bathing has been found to lower blood pressure, heart rate, and levels of stress hormones (Li 2010).

The terpenes in volatile oils released by the forest plant community have natural antimicrobial and insecticidal qualities that protect trees from germs and parasites. A tree emits these active substances to create a field of protection around itself. The most common compounds in these volatile oils are α-pinene, d-limonene, β-pinene, sabinene, myrcene, and camphene.

Clinical research on these oils shows that they possess a range of pharmacological effects that can benefit the human body as well. They evoke a well-demonstrated immune response that increases natural killer cell activity, an effect that can last for days. Many forest terpenes normalize inflammation and reduce oxidative stress. They promote relaxation and lower nervous system activity in general. The lifting of mood that many people experience in nature is partially due to a reduction in cortisol levels; β-pinene has antidepressive properties and α-pinene may enhance sleep (Antonelli et al. 2020).

Ecology of Sesquiterpene Lactones

As an example of the rich gamut of ecological relationships that terpenes are involved in, consider the sesquiterpene lactones. Many flowering plants contain these active molecules, which play a pivotal role in facilitating the plants' integration with their community, such as the complexities of their life in the soil.

Rooted plants don't move, making them easy targets, compounded by the inability to avoid bad climate, all of which may affect their resistance to infections. Thus plants are capable of producing a range of chemicals that help them withstand attack from fungi, bacteria, and viruses. Typically, these compounds take the form of alkaloids, phenolics, and terpenoids. In the sunflower family especially, sesquiterpene lactones are one of the main mechanisms for this defense. Sesquiterpenes can cause disruption of a microbe's cell membrane, leading to cell death. They also fulfill a wide range of other functions in plants, such as the compounds that deter herbivores or, conversely, attract pest predators, those that protect against damage from UV light and ozone, and those that function as hormones or allelochemicals.

While sesquiterpene lactones are produced by plants for the benefit of not people but the plants themselves, they are nevertheless of great importance in herbal medicine. Herbs that contain pharmacologically active sesquiterpene lactones have a central role in the materia medicas of the world. They are known to contribute to the treatment of cardiovascular diseases, function as antimalarials, inhibit tumor growth and development, help prevent neurodegeneration, and express antimigraine, analgesic, and sedative activities.

Perhaps the most recognizable feature is the group's bitter flavor. Sesquiterpene lactones provide the characteristic bitterness to vegetables such as chicory, where it is considered a positive, but also to lettuce, where it is considered a negative. Thanks to their sesquiterpene lactone content, some herbs, too, are bitter-tasting, and they are used in many cultures to support upper digestive system activity, though there is no consensus regarding the mechanism by which the chemosensory stimulation of bitter taste receptors could enhance digestion.

Mycorrhizae: Synergy in the Soil

The soil is home to one of the most important and unique synergistic relationships known: mycorrhizae. A mycorrhiza is a unique symbiotic association between soil-borne fungi and a plant. The fungi colonize the plant's roots; among other benefits, this arrangement increases the plant's ability to absorb water and nutrients, while the plant provides the fungi with carbohydrates formed from photosynthesis. Plants can allocate up to 30 percent of the carbon made available through photosynthesis to mycorrhizal fungi, and in return, the fungi can acquire up to 80 percent of the phosphorus and nitrogen a plant needs.

This ubiquitous symbiosis between plants and fungi is the basis of life on land and an insightful example of symbiogenesis. The fossil record shows that plants first began to settle on dry land some four hundred million years ago. These plants lacked roots, relying on their association with fungi for the uptake of water and minerals (Remy et al. 1994). That early symbiosis played a crucial role in the evolution of vascular plants. Today, we see mycorrhizal associations in about 90 percent of all plants, including ferns and mosses (Brundrett 2002).

Arbuscular Mycorrhizal Fungi

The most common type of fungi that colonize plant roots in a mutualistic symbiosis are classified as arbuscular mycorrhizal fungi (AMF). Filaments of their mycelium actually grow into the cells of the symbiont plant, producing highly branched structures called arbuscules ("little trees"), inside the cell walls but outside the plasma membranes. The plasma membrane of a plant cell becomes wrapped around the arbuscule, providing lots of surface area for the exchange of nutrients and information between plant and fungus. The arbuscules last only a few days before they are dissolved and digested by the host plant, so they are constantly growing and dissolving in the roots of a plant with this type of mycorrhiza (Luginbuehl and Oldroyd 2017).

Only a small number of AMF are known, somewhere in the range of 240 species. But AMF species are not host-specific; they are able to colonize multiple species of plants, and plant roots tend to be colonized by a number of fungi species. The fungi form extensive underground networks, composed of hyphae (mycelial filaments) and spores, connecting plants of different species and even different ecosystems. These networks represent significant underground "nutrient highways" that benefit entire plant and microbial communities (Bonfante and Genre 2010). One plant may provide the carbon for the establishment of the mycelial network that another plant of a different species can utilize for mineral uptake (Lanfranco, Bonfante, and Genre 2016; Simard et al. 1997).

The whole matrix of life on land is a result of this mycorrhizal symbiosis, suggesting that there is more going on than nutrient exchange.

Secondary Metabolites in Mycorrhizal Networks

Every organism on Earth relies on associations with its neighbors to sustain life, and these associations are facilitated by chemical cues. In the rhizosphere, which includes plant roots and the surrounding area of soil influenced by the roots, plants exude chemicals to effectively communicate with their neighboring soil organisms—and they do so in (relatively) enormous volume. As it turns out, the rhizosphere has a dynamic chemical ecology.

The compounds released by plant roots include both primary and secondary metabolites. The soil in direct contact with plant roots represents a particularly rich environment for microbes, and these plant metabolites have direct effects on microbial communities, especially mycorrhizal networks. Flavonoids, for example, stimulate or inhibit microbial gene expression, attract beneficial soil bacteria toward the roots, inhibit root pathogens, and stimulate mycorrhizal spore germination (Hassan and Mathesius 2012).

As an example, the invasion of plant roots by mycorrhizal hyphae is a complex and tightly controlled process that itself depends on diverse secondary metabolites. Mycorrhizal fungi occur among many other inhabitants of the soil, and successful development of the plant-fungi symbioses relies on a signal exchange that allows mutual recognition and reprogramming for the anticipated physical interaction. The plant roots secrete secondary metabolites known as strigolactones. When the fungi perceive these strigolactones, they respond by producing their own signaling molecules for the plant (Mailett et al. 2011). The strigolactones appear to stimulate branching and growth of fungal hyphae, facilitating the establishment of a symbiotic relationship between plant and fungus.

Termite-Fungi Symbiosis

Complex symbiotic relationships like those of mycorrhizal networks seem to be characteristic throughout ecosystems. As an example, signaling metabolites similar to plant-root strigolactones facilitate a unique symbiosis between some termites and fungi. Much like farmers growing crops, the termites cultivate the fungi for food. And they've been doing so for an incredible length of time: Fossil evidence suggests that the termite and fungal species coevolved at least thirty million years ago.

The termites cultivate the fungi in structures called combs. Foraging workers gather woody material, chew it up, and swallow it. Upon returning to the nest, they evacuate this material as pseudofeces, passing it on to nest workers, who mold it into the fungus comb. The woody slurry is inoculated with fungal spores that germinate and spread hyphae through the comb. As these grow, they digest cellulose, converting it to simpler sugars and nitrogen. The termites then eat the enriched food. A colony generally has a large number of fungus combs, gathered into a series of galleries atop the nest called a fungus garden. And an array of 375 different secondary metabolites have been found to characterize the termite-fungi interaction, including sesquiterpenes and other volatile terpenes.

Ecology of Aroma:
Biogenic Volatile Organic Compounds

Almost all plants emit a wide range of volatile chemicals, known technically as biogenic volatile organic compounds (BVOCs). (Calling them BVOCs emphasizes their natural origins, as opposed to the VOCS—volatile organic compounds—emitted by industrial technology and human life in general.) BVOCs are the compounds that give plants (and their essential oils) their characteristic aromas.

Analysis techniques such as gas chromatography and mass spectrometry can be used to identify the exact molecules responsible for aromas, whether we're talking about the scent of a single flower or that of an entire ecosystem, like the tropical rainforest. As it turns out, many of the BVOCs that give plants their unique aromas are the same secondary metabolites through which plants cultivate their ecological relationships.

As noted in the earlier discussion of mycorrhizae, secondary metabolites play a key role in the soil, where they are central to a plant's interactions with microbes and other plants. That multifaceted metabolite-driven ecological matrix rises from the rhizosphere to the atmosphere.

Consider the example of sesquiterpenes. These secondary metabolites are deeply involved in a plant's ecological relationships, facilitating its integration with mycorrhizae and other aspects of its community. Sesquiterpenes also comprise a major part of a plant's BVOCs. For instance, β-caryophyllene has been detected in 50 to 70 percent of flower aromas of all plants studied.

Among other things, plants use sesquiterpenes to protect their aboveground parts from ozone. Ozone, produced by the action of UV radiation on oxygen, is a natural part of Earth's atmosphere, but it is also a powerful oxidant, entering plant leaf stomata (pores) and oxidizing (burning) tissues within. However, the intracellular spaces within leaves where the ozone might diffuse are the same spaces where sesquiterpenes accumulate. Here, the sesquiterpenes act as antioxidants, defending plants from ozone damage. As each plant and all its neighbors release sesquiterpenes and other volatile compounds, they contribute to the aroma of the habitat at large.

In any ecosystem, much more is going on than the responses of individuals. In nature, plants rarely occur as isolated specimens; instead, they are members of communities in which they compete for resources, exchange information with other plants and organisms, and, sometimes, assist their neighbors.

Attractants and Repellents

The whole range of a plant's volatile terpenes are found in its leaves and flowering tops. Their ready availability to other organisms, like insects, animals, and humans, suggests that they play a role in many different interactions.

At the level of the ecosystem, BVOCs often serve as modulators, working to promote balance between the needs of different species. When a plant has been damaged by herbivores, it might begin to produce volatiles that attract the natural predators of those herbivores, thus minimizing the potential damage the herbivores can inflict on the plant's local habitat (Kessler and Baldwin 2001; War et al. 2011). When attacked by insects, a plant can release BVOCs that induce nearby plants to produce protective volatiles for themselves, such as compounds that repel female insects from laying eggs, or it may change the proportions of compounds in its normal BVOC mixture to repel the insects directly (Unsicker, Kunert, and Gershenzon 2009). If infected with fungi, bacteria, or a virus, a plant releases volatiles that not only have direct antimicrobial effects but also trigger systemic resistance in uninfected parts of the plant and in neighboring plants (Hammerbacher, Coutinho, and Gershenzon 2019).

BVOCs are crucial to the dynamics of pollination. These volatiles, released from leaves, flowers, and fruits into the atmosphere and from roots into the soil, provide a reproductive advantage by attracting pollinators and seed dispersers (Shuttleworth and Johnson 2009). In some cases, a plant's scent can serve as a "private channel" to lure a specific pollinator species (Chen et al. 2009). Some researchers have reported that floral scent functions as an important attractant in the specialized pollination system of spider wasps within the genus *Hemipepsis*.

The attractant-repellent dynamic governed by BVOCs extends beyond pollination, of course, in ways unique to the particular ecological need. For example, some sesquiterpenes are extremely bitter and repel birds from devouring certain plants. At the same time, other sesquiterpenes actually attract birds, such as α-farnesene, which is responsible for the characteristic smell of apples, thus aiding the spread of seeds.

Starlings, Tits, and Nest Building

A fascinating role of these volatile constituents is their involvement in the selection of nesting material by passerine birds. Passerines comprise more than half of the world's bird species and include all the songbirds, sparrows, and finches. Researchers have observed European starlings blending fresh herbs, usually aromatic species like cow parsley, elderflower, hogweed, and yarrow, into their dry nest material (Gwinner 2012). Similarly, Corsican blue tits have been seen using up to five different aromatic herbs in their nests (Lambrechts and Santos 2000). Why are these birds using specific aromatic herbs in this way? Research found that birds with aromatic herbs in their nest material were more likely to spend time in their nests, showed better behavior toward their eggs, and became active earlier in the day. Fledglings from nests with the herbs had a greater body mass and were overall healthier, with fewer mites.

Sesquiterpenes and other BVOCs present in the herb material, the researchers theorized, repel parasites and also mask the chemical cues that parasites use to find a host. The leaves may be warming and insulating. In the case of the starlings, the volatiles were shown to be sedating to the parent bird. Some of the BVOCs identified from nest air samples included limonene and caryophyllene.

Cloud Formation

Perhaps most unexpected is the fundamental involvement of BVOCs in the formation of clouds. Clouds consist of ice or liquid water droplets light enough to stay suspended in the atmosphere. When the air becomes saturated with water, the vapor condenses on extremely small particles known as cloud seeds. As more vapor condenses, the particles grow in size, forming droplets visible in the sky as clouds. If cloud droplets become heavy enough, they fall to the ground as rain. A typical raindrop is about 2 millimeters in diameter, a typical cloud droplet is about 0.02 millimeter, and a typical cloud seed is on the order of 0.0001 millimeter.

Most condensation nuclei are produced by natural and man-made fires on land and wave action over the oceans. Dust and sulfate from volcanic activity can be a major source, as can dust and soil particles blown into the atmosphere. However, another major contributing source is molecules formed by the oxidation of BVOCs released by plants, and especially those in forests (Hartz et al. 2005).

The countless trees of the Amazon rainforest naturally emit these compounds, including terpene and isoprene. They are swept into the upper atmosphere by cloud convection, reaching as high as 15,000 meters, where the extremely cold temperature (about −55 degrees Celsius) facilitates particle formation. Wind speeds at this level of the upper atmosphere are high, and so these particles and the clouds they form are redistributed around the planet (Loreto et al. 2013).

Whether BVOCs are just by-products of various plant processes or actively produced and used as a sophisticated language by plants to have a dialogue with other organisms is, as yet, not able to be known. What we do know is that these chemical signals are firmly embedded in the ecological dynamics of the world, from deep Earth to the high atmosphere, including everything in between—such as humans.

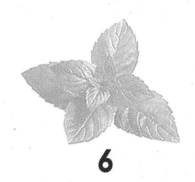

6

The Pharmacology of Herbal Synergy

The ecological insights discussed in the previous chapter illuminate an exquisitely complex pattern of chemical interactions. To explore the mechanisms of these interactions as they play out in the field of human health care, we must delve into pharmacology, the study of therapeutic substances in all their aspects.

Therapeutic substances are usually called drugs, but this term can cause some confusion when considering herbal medicines, as there is a tendency to differentiate between the categories of herbs and drugs. It is worth noting that the word *drug* is derived from the Old English *drogge*, first recorded in the fourteenth century, which designated any substance used in the composition or preparation of medicines. *Drogge*, in turn, is thought to come from the Old Dutch *droge*, "dry," which was used in terms such as *droge-vate*, "dry barrels," or *droge waere*, "dry wares." These "dry wares" were specifically dried herbs and spices—the medicines of that era. Thus our modern word *drug* relates to the use of dried plants in medicine. *Drug* is an herbal word.

As we have seen, modern theory is starting to recognize that ideas long considered flaws in herbal medicine—like relying on synergistic and holistic therapies rather than the "one disease–one target–one drug" treatments that have dominated Western medicine—are becoming cutting-edge concepts. In this chapter, we'll focus on the pharmacology of herbal synergy and the mechanisms by which it works.

Putting it in the most basic of terms, the treatment of health disorders with herbal medicines involves active secondary metabolites of low molecular weight and of great structural diversity that have a range of pharmacological effects. Given the chemical nature of the interactions between herbs and humans, it should be no surprise that the mechanisms of herbal activity can be explored, examined, and potentially explained through the lens of pharmacology.

Pharmacological Synergy in Herbal Medicines

Pharmacological synergy is a common characteristic in herbs used medicinally. This synergism may result from one constituent enhancing the therapeutic effect of another by regulating its absorption and metabolism. For example, in ginseng, saponins may increase the absorption of corticosteroids, and in St. John's wort, hyperoside increases the solubility of hypericin (He et al. 2020).

Another model of synergy would be plants in which certain constituents potentiate the effects of others. Goldenseal (*Hydrastis canadensis*), for example, is typically used as an antimicrobial and for relief of gastrointestinal symptoms. Cooperative interaction occurs between its constituent berberine, an antimicrobial alkaloid, and a number of its flavonoids. Though the flavonoids have no antibacterial activity on their own, they have been shown to increase the activity of berberine. In other words, they potentiate berberine's effects—a clear example of synergy, where the combined action of the two constituents is greater than the sum of the parts (Junio et al. 2011).

These same kinds of synergistic interactions carry forward into formulations that employ multiple herbs. In these cases, the pharmacological activities of one herb might be potentiated, prolonged, or (in the case of adverse effects) reduced by the other herbs in the formula. In traditional use, such combinations appear to effect a more favorable response than the "active" herb used alone, which suggests that the therapeutic effects of these medicines may arise from the synergistic actions of herb constituents.

Modes of Action of Secondary Metabolites

Secondary metabolites have been central to science's discoveries at the level of cellular biology. Using small-molecule probes that interact with specific proteins has opened the exploration of the role proteins play in cells. These small-molecule probes are often plant secondary metabolites (Carlson 2010). So what has been discovered that can illuminate our understanding of the mechanisms that underlie herbal medicine?

In the material that follows, we'll explore a small selection of molecular-scale mechanisms from an herbal perspective, followed by a look at some general processes. The most widespread secondary metabolites, such as the flavonoids and terpenes commonly found in essential oils, have multitarget effects, modulating the activity of proteins, nucleic acids, and cell membranes (Dixon et al. 2007). Remember, though, that often the observed effects of an herb or an herbal formula cannot be pinpointed to a single secondary metabolite. They manifest due to the synergistic interactions of several constituents and, for this reason, can target a broad spectrum of imbalances.

Modification of Proteins and DNA Bases

Although proteins were once thought to act as discrete entities, performing their functions without significant cross talk with other macromolecules, today it is widely recognized that proteins function through a complex network of biomolecule interactions, the so-called interactome.

Proteins are the primary structural and functional molecules in the cell and are made up of chains of amino acids. These chains are folded into secondary and tertiary structures to form the characteristic shape of functional protein. Proteins are constantly changing to meet the needs of the cell. Among many other functions, they often act as enzymes and receptors.

The most abundant targets for secondary metabolites are proteins. Secondary metabolites that form bonds with proteins induce a conformational (three-dimensional) transformation, changing the biological activity of the proteins.

Interactions with Cell Membranes

All living cells are surrounded by a membrane that acts as a barrier between that which is inside and that which is outside. This membrane houses a multitude of proteins, such as receptors, enabling communication or the exchange of substances with other cells or tissues. Many fat-soluble secondary metabolites easily bind to the inner layer of the membrane. For example, the terpenes in essential oils assemble in membranes and can change membrane fluidity and increase permeability, an important factor in their antimicrobial effects. The same terpenes modulate the activity of calcium channels; this is, as an example, considered to be the basis of the relaxing effects of peppermint oil on smooth muscles in the intestines.

Facilitation of Cell Communication

Cell signaling is part of a complex system of communication that governs the basic activities of cells and coordinates cell actions. This ability of cells to perceive and respond to information is the basis for physiological development, repair, and immunity as well as normal homeostasis.

These cell signals are chemical and take the form of signaling molecules. A signaling molecule binding with a receptor on a cell surface triggers a cascade of events that carries the signal to the cell interior. Different receptors are specific for different molecules. Once a receptor protein receives a signal, it undergoes a conformational change, which in turn launches a series of biochemical reactions within the cell, called signal transduction cascades, eventually eliciting a response.

Secondary metabolites are among the signaling molecules that dock with cellular receptors and initiate these signal transduction cascades.

As discussed in chapter 1, plants and animals, including humans, came to exist in a coevolutionary context, developing over deep time in an intimate ecological dynamic that has yielded significant dependence and cooperation across species. The secondary metabolites found in plants, including the herbs used medicinally, have been shaped by evolution to interact with human proteins and thus can induce conformational changes and bring about a modification of their bioactivity. In fact, they have the ability to modulate more than one molecular target; thus, additive and synergistic activities occur (Wink and Schimmer 2010).

Drug Development and Discovery

Plants have evolved and adapted over millions of years to survive and thrive in the context of often challenging ecologies. Their successful use by traditional healers has often led researchers to identify them as potential sources of new pharmaceutical drugs.

According to one estimate, half of the medications approved in North America from 1981 through 2010 have natural origins. More followed, and today a considerable number of natural products and compounds derived from them are currently in clinical trials (Butler, Robertson, and Cooper 2014; Newman and Cragg 2016). According to the World Health Organization, 80 percent of people still rely on plant-based traditional medicines for primary health care.

The U.S. National Cancer Institute (NCI) has identified more than three thousand plants from which anticancer drugs are or could be made, including ginseng, Madagascar periwinkle, mayapple, and western yew. Thanks to two drugs derived from the Madagascar's rosy periwinkle, the likelihood of remission for a child suffering from leukemia increased by 85 percent between 1960 and 1997.

The International Union for the Conservation of Nature estimates that between fifty thousand and eighty thousand flowering plants are used medicinally worldwide. Since less than 10 percent of the world's biodiversity has been evaluated for potential biological activity, many more useful natural compounds await discovery. Yet out of this tiny portion have come a surprising number of prescription medicines.

From this, we can see that the contribution of plants to the cutting edge of new drug development is profound. This is especially the case for those impacting the human immune response, a direct consequence of coevolution. Textbooks on drug development are replete with examples of the natural roots of modern drugs, but there are some unusual and surprising case studies. One key insight is the breadth and depth of functions exhibited by secondary metabolites. It seems that natural selection favors metabolites that are versatile and multitargeted, and among plant constituents, secondary metabolites have been the most successful source of these new drug leads (Dias, Urban, and Roessner 2012).

Aspirin
Probably the most well-known example of a pharmaceutical drug with herbal origins is acetylsalicylic acid, or aspirin, as discussed in chapter 3 (page 61). This chemical is not found in nature and so must be manufactured industrially. The manufacturing process utilized a molecule that is found in plants as its raw material. Thus aspirin is derived from salicin isolated from the bark of the willow tree (*Salix alba*).

Heroin and Codeine
The effects of the opium poppy (*Papaver somniferum*) led to the investigation of opium for its "active" constituents, and morphine was identified in 1803. Chemically modifying crude morphine produces heroin, which in turn can be readily converted to codeine.

Cardiac Glycosides
Foxglove (*Digitalis purpurea*) is the source of a number of cardiac glycosides, including the digoxin and digitoxin, both used today as medications for the treatment of heart conditions. These secondary metabolites enhance the strength of cardiac contractibility, alleviating the symptoms of heart failure. Digitoxin and its analogues have long been used in the management of congestive heart failure.

Taxol

Paclitaxel (Taxol) is a complex diterpenoid isolated originally from the bark of the Pacific yew tree (*Taxus brevifolia*). It is a mitotic inhibitor used in cancer chemotherapy. In 1962, the USDA first collected the bark as part of its exploratory plant screening program at the National Cancer Institute. The extraction of just one gram of paclitaxel requires the bark from about three mature hundred-year-old trees. However, the daily dose is in the range of two grams. Current demand for paclitaxel is in the region of one hundred to two hundred kilograms yearly (i.e., fifty thousand treatments), and so it is now produced synthetically (Dias, Urban, and Roessner 2012).

Cyclosporin

Cyclosporin is a drug used in organ transplantation as an immunosuppressant to prevent rejection. It reduces the activity of the immune system by interfering with the activity and growth of T cells. It was initially isolated from a fungus found in a soil sample obtained in 1969 from Hardangervidda, Norway. Interestingly, it is a close relative of the important medicinal fungi cordyceps (*Cordyceps* spp.) (Svarstad, Bugge, and Dhillion 2000).

Tamiflu

In 2006, a global bird flu pandemic was thought to be impending, though thankfully it did not occur. In the face of this, medical authorities ranging from the World Health Organization (WHO) and the U.S. Centers for Disease Control and Prevention (CDC) to family practitioners proposed the oral antiviral Tamiflu (oseltamivir) as the drug of choice. Not only was it being prescribed in unprecedented volume, it was also being stockpiled by many countries in the event of the worst-case scenario.

Tamiflu interferes with the attachment of viruses to the surface of cells, thus blocking the infection. At the time, Tamiflu was manufactured from shikimic acid, a molecule extracted from the fruits of Chinese star anise. Shikimic acid is used as a convenient building block for the drug, not because it has any antiviral activity. The great demand for it, combined with crop failure (which could be seen as early signs of climate change), led to major concerns about Tamiflu supplies.

Emodin

Emodin is a polyphenol from the anthraquinone family. It is widely distributed in plants and is found in many traditional medicinal herbs, such as aloe, buckthorn, Chinese rhubarb (*Rheum palmatum*), and senna. It is also produced by many species of fungi, including those of the *Cortinarius* genus, with more than two thousand species; the characteristic rust brown to brownish-red color of the mushroom and its spores is due to the presence of emodin and related molecules.

The ecological importance of emodin can be seen in its presence in seventeen plant families from around the world. It is involved in plant-plant, plant-animal, and plant-soil interactions. It inhibits the growth of roots and shoots of sunflowers and corn. It has a feeding-deterrent effect on a large spectrum of organisms, from invertebrates to vertebrates.

Although it was first described more than seventy-five years ago, many of its biological properties have only recently been discovered. Primarily known for its stimulant laxative action, emodin possesses a wide spectrum of pharmacological properties, including anticancer, liver protection, anti-inflammatory, antioxidant, and antimicrobial activities. It affects the immune system, vasomotor system, and metabolic processes (Dong et al. 2016). Research has found that emodin can inhibit infection with and replication of a number of viruses, including herpes simplex types 1 and 2, human cytomegalovirus, Epstein-Barr, coxsackievirus B, hepatitis B, influenza A, SARS-CoV, dengue, and Zika virus (Shao et al. 2022).

That a single molecule can have such a range of effects is still controversial, but this multifunctionality is a common phenomenon among secondary metabolites. As we have seen, these metabolites play many roles in the complexities of nature. Their evolution as an integral part of the diverse interactions between plants, animals, and their environment might explain their pharmacological multifunctionality.

Metformin

A fascinating but often overlooked example of a medication derived from plants is the antidiabetic drug metformin. The American Diabetes Association recommends metformin for newly diagnosed patients with non-insulin-dependent (type 2) diabetes, before they try other drugs. It was the third top drug prescribed in 2020, with more than ninety-two million prescriptions in the United States alone. In fact, so much metformin is taken in the United States that a recent study found higher trace levels of it (presumably from the urine of people taking it) in Lake Michigan than of any other drug, including caffeine.

According to the CDC, about 9 percent of the U.S. population experience type 2 diabetes, which is preventable through appropriate diet, regular physical activity, and weight loss. It can be controlled with these same activities, but medication is often prescribed. Type 2 diabetes is partly due to insulin resistance, an inability to lower blood glucose levels in response to the hormone insulin. Metformin works as an insulin sensitizer, helping to restore the body's ability to respond to insulin, while most other drug medications increase the amount of insulin the body produces.

The European herb goat's rue (*Galega officinalis*) has been used since the Middle Ages to treat diabetic symptoms. In the early twentieth century, researchers isolated a compound from it, called guanidine, that could lower blood glucose levels in animals but was also toxic. It was made more tolerable by bonding two guanidines together, forming a molecule called a biguanide. Metformin is one such form of biguanide, first synthesized in 1929 and marketed in the late 1950s under the trade name Glucophage ("glucose eater"). Metformin helps control the amount of glucose in the blood, decreasing the amount of glucose absorbed from food and the amount of glucose made by the liver. It also increases responsiveness to insulin.

However, it appears to have some other surprising properties. Some people take metformin because they believe it may have an impact in promoting general health and slowing the aging process. In one often-quoted study, diabetic patients taking metformin lived longer than diabetic patients not taking it—and also longer than people without diabetes (Bannister et al. 2014).

A specific trial, called the Targeting Aging with Metformin (TAME) trial, to test metformin as an anti-aging molecule was initiated in 2018. The results are yet to be published, but if they are positive, metformin will probably be the medication approved by the FDA for this type of prevention (Prattichizzo et al. 2018).

Artemisinin, Sweet Annie, and the Nobel Prize

The Nobel Prize–winning development of successful treatments for malaria demonstrates the potential when ancient traditional herbal techniques are applied in pharmacologically sound and politically relevant ways.

Malaria is a devastating disease affecting millions of people across Asia and Africa each year. It is caused by the single-celled *Plasmodium* parasite and spread by the *Anopheles* mosquito. It has long had serious effects on both mortality rates and quality of life, and in turn on the economic and social fabric of nations and societies. Various methods have been utilized to mitigate its frequency and effects, but this has proven to be a never-ending battle requiring constant attention. In 2021, the WHO estimated there were 247 million cases of malaria, with an estimated 619,000 deaths globally. Most of the cases and the deaths occurred in Africa and affected primarily children and pregnant women. Children under the age of five accounted for 80 percent of all African malaria deaths (WHO 2022).

The development of malarial chemotherapy is intimately linked with the history of herbal febrifuges. In 1820, French scientists discovered quinine, the first antimalarial drug, in the bark of cinchona trees (*Cinchona* spp.). Cinchona was used medicinally by the Inca and had been introduced to Europe in the 1700s. From this came chloroquine, the antimalarial of the past century.

Although plant-based quinine medicines have been fundamental to the treatment of malaria, all have lost effectiveness over time due to the development of resistance. In traditional practice, often several plants are used in combination, which protects against resistance. Well over a thousand plants have been used traditionally for the treatment of malaria (Willcox et al. 2004).

The current antimalarial drug of choice is artemisinin, a sesquiterpene alkaloid that was first discovered in 1972 in the leaves of the Chinese herb qinghao, known as sweet Annie in North America and botanically as *Artemisia annua*. For her discovery of artemisinin, Dr. Tu Youyou received the 2015 Nobel Prize in Medicine. Artemisinin can be used as an antimalarial, anticancer, and anti-inflammatory agent. Its derivatives also possess anthelmintic, fungicidal, and antiviral properties.

Qinghao has long been used in China; it was first noted in a document dating from 168 BCE, while the first record of its use for malaria comes from 341 CE. In the mid-1960s, early in the Cultural Revolution and during the Vietnam War, China responded to requests from North Vietnam for help in treating malaria. This led to the exploration of the extensive traditional medicine pharmacopoeia with modern pharmaceutical chemistry and, hence, the discovery of the antimalarial properties of extracts of the leaves of *Artemisia annua*. The process of identifying the antimalarial constituents, their structures and properties, and their antimalarial activities involved botany, ethnobotany, phytochemistry, pharmacology, traditional Chinese medicine, Western medicine, agronomy, and a gamut of issues relating to manufacture and commercialization.

The question arises: Is the effect of whole plant extract simply the effect of the isolated active constituents? As it turns out, a tea made of whole-plant qinghao has greater in vitro and in vivo antimalarial activity than isolated constituents at an equivalent dose. But the amount of artemisinin contained in a traditionally prepared tea is small compared to the recommended dose. The effectiveness of the preparation can be attributed to the presence of other compounds in *A. annua*, especially flavonoids, which act synergistically to enhance the action of artemisinin. In addition to at least forty-six flavonoids, *A. annua* also contains phenolic compounds, including coumarins and phenolic acids, and the contribution of all of these in combination may be important for anti-malarial efficacy (Ferreira et al. 2010).

As we've seen, some compounds in plants can work synergistically to dramatically affect the bioavailability and metabolism of bioactive constituents. In the case of the artemisinin in *A. annua*, there are many possible synergistic mechanisms; other constituents may increase the permeability of the plasmodium membrane, for example, or improve the absorption of artemisinin.

Although *A. annua* has been used for several thousand years, resistance does not seem to have appeared. Resistance to isolated artemisinin has been detected.

Today, the use of teas prepared from the dried leaves of locally grown *A. annua* is being promoted as an alternative treatment for malaria in areas where people do not have access to or cannot afford effective antimalarials such as artemisinin combination therapy.

One factor that has not been extensively exploited in conventional antimalarial therapy is the synergistic interaction of multiherb formulations. Traditional formulations for malaria typically include not only *A. annua* but also several hepatoprotective plants, such as licorice and ginger. Ginger may be commonly used in traditional antimalarial formulations because nausea and vomiting are common symptoms of the disease; there is good clinical evidence for the antiemetic effect of ginger especially in pregnancy, although it has not specifically been tested for its antiemetic effect in the context of malaria.

The Pharmacological Basis of Herbal Activity

The insights gained from the technology that is now available, informed by an ever-growing respect for traditional methods, is leading to a cornucopia of pharmacological insights. The following examples explore the mechanisms underlying some specific clinically relevant herbal treatments.

Snowdrop, Sage, and Dementia

Dementia is a clinical syndrome wherein a person experiences gradual decline of mental and cognitive capabilities. As the disease progresses, the patient's ability to function independently deteriorates due to memory loss.

Neurotransmitters facilitate the transmission of electrical signals between a neuron and another cell. There are a number of them, including glutamate, gamma-aminobutyric acid (GABA), and acetylcholine. Acetylcholine is deeply involved with attention and memory. Reduced acetylcholine levels are found in various forms of dementia, leading to the development of therapeutic approaches aimed at facilitating what is called "cholinergic replacement."

However, if taken as a medication, acetylcholine is quickly inactivated; enzymes in the blood work rapidly to break it down. This means that treatment must employ other methods to achieve a meaningful elevation in a patient's acetylcholine levels. One approach has been to target acetylcholinesterase, the enzyme responsible for the breakdown of acetylcholine. Inhibiting the activity of the enzyme helps maintain existing levels of acetylcholine. For this reason, acetylcholinesterase inhibitors are used as a treatment for various dementias, potentially stabilizing or improving cognition, mood, and behavior in patients. Unfortunately, as diseases like Alzheimer's progress, there are fewer and fewer intact cholinergic neurons and so there is less potential for this approach to work. Thus this treatment only slows the symptomatic progression of the disease and doesn't alter the underlying disease process.

Acetylcholinesterase Inhibitors in Plants

Around the world, medicinal plants have long been used for treating dementia. They are generally herbs with known anti-inflammatory and antioxidant activity associated with neuroprotective effects.

Some plants contain precisely the type of acetylcholinesterase inhibitors needed. Physostigmine, from the Calabar bean (*Physostigma venenosum*), was the first to be used clinically, but acetylcholinesterase inhibitors are now known to be widely found in plants. One example is huperzine A, an alkaloid from a club moss (*Huperzia serrata*) that grows in moist, hilly regions in southern China. Huperzine A has been shown to be an active acetylcholinesterase inhibitor. The club moss itself is a component of a traditional tea formula for the elderly. Another example is galantamine, a drug (trade name Razadyne) prescribed for the treatment of mild to moderate dementia. It is an alkaloid first discovered and isolated from the bulbs of snowdrop (*Galanthus* spp.) by Bulgarian chemists in 1956. Galantamine is an effective acetylcholinesterase inhibitor, and at the same time it reduces damaging cellular oxidative stress (Tewari et al. 2018).

European folk herbalism has a long tradition of using well-known herbs such as lemon balm, rosemary, sage, and thyme for treating dementia. Several of these plants have been investigated for their memory-enhancing activity and have yielded compounds that may be of clinical relevance in Alzheimer's management.

In *The British Herbal* (1756), John Hill wrote of sage that it "will retard that rapid progress of decay that treads upon our heels so fast in latter years of life, will preserve faculties and memory more valuable to the rational mind than life itself." Recent research has gone a long way to substantiate such historical use of sage for memory enhancement, as anti-acetylcholinesterase activity has been found in both sage essential oil and extract (Lopresti 2017). This could account, at least in part, for its memory-enhancing reputation. The Latin name for the sage genus is *Salvia* and comes from the Latin *salvare*, meaning "to be saved." *Salvia* (with more than seven hundred species) is the largest genus in the mint family, and though not all have been researched pharmacologically, many have actions on the central nervous system (CNS). The genus features prominently in the pharmacopoeias of many countries throughout the world. European sage and Chinese sage have been widely investigated phytochemically and a vast array of biological activities have been identified, many of which are relevant to CNS disorders.

Free radical damage has been described in the pathological changes that occur in Alzheimer's, and so the use of antioxidants, which combat this damage, is considered an important therapeutic strategy. Research has shown that sage exhibits both antioxidant and anti-inflammatory properties, which implies that its memory-enhancing reputation may be due to a combination of actions (Margetts et al. 2022).

In many cases, the effects of these phytochemicals on the human CNS might be linked either to their ecological roles in the life of the plant or to molecular and biochemical similarities between the biology of plants and that of higher animals (Kennedy and Wightman 2011).

Cannabinoids and the Endocannabinoid System

Health is not static but rather a dynamic state, which differs under various circumstances. Instead of trying to attain a perfect state of health, our preventive and therapeutic approaches should rather aim for increasing our ability to adapt. Herbalism is uniquely poised to support the inherent capacity of the body to respond to the pressures of life in such a way that it augments resilience to illness, supporting homeostasis and integration.

We've talked about the ways in which the exploration of secondary metabolites has opened the door to new understandings of the body's systems and structures. A recent and unexpected example is that of the endocannabinoid system, illuminating the physiology of integration, homeostasis, and the value of well-being.

Though the efficacy of cannabis has long been well established, until recently there was no understanding of the mechanisms that enabled it to reduce nausea, quell seizures, relieve pain, improve sleep, and stimulate appetite. It is now known that cannabis is able to elicit its effects via its cannabinoids—that is, compounds that bind with the human endocannabinoid system (ECS).

The human cannabinoid receptor known as CB1 was discovered in 1990, and rapidly followed by CB2. The discovery of these receptors resulted in the uncovering of the naturally occurring neurotransmitters called endocannabinoids—that is, cannabinoids made in the human body (*endo* means "within," as in "within the body") (Pertwee 2006). There are two major endocannabinoids: anandamide and 2-arachidonoylglycerol (2-AG).

Phytocannabinoids are plant substances that interact with human cannabinoid receptors. In cannabis, tetrahydrocannabinol (THC) is the primary psychoactive cannabinoid, but other cannabinoids such as cannabidiol (CBD) and cannabinol (CBN) have a variety of properties.

Studying phyto- and endocannabinoids led researchers to identify the ECS as a previously unknown molecular signaling system within the body. It performs multiple tasks, working toward maintaining a stable environment (homeostasis) despite fluctuations in the external environment. When an imbalance is detected within our internal environment, the body synthesizes endocannabinoids that interact with the cannabinoid receptors. This stimulates a chemical response that works to return the physiological process back to homeostasis. The endocannabinoid system has emerged as an important modulator of both emotional and non-emotional behaviors (Micale and Drago 2018).

The endogenous cannabinoid system, or endocannabinoid system, is perhaps the most important physiologic system involved in establishing and maintaining human health. Endocannabinoids and their receptors are found in each tissue of the body and perform different tasks, but the goal is always the same: homeostasis (Hillard 2015).

Homeostasis is best described as the ability to maintain stable internal conditions that are necessary for survival. Homeostatic balance is pivotal in all life processes, so the ECS appears to be involved in just about everything. Among the many things the ECS regulates, consider gastrointestinal activity, activity of the heart and blood vessels, pain perception, maintenance of bone mass, protection of neurons, hormonal regulation, metabolism control, immune function, inflammatory reactions, and inhibition of tumor cells.

There are two main cannabinoid receptors: CB1 and CB2. CB1 receptors predominate in the nervous system, connective tissues, gonads, glands, and organs, whereas CB2 receptors are more abundant outside the nervous system, especially in the immune system. However, both types are found throughout the body.

Endocannabinoids are found at the intersection of the body's various systems, allowing communication and coordination between different cell types. At the site of an injury, for example, cannabinoids can be found decreasing the release of activators and sensitizers from the injured tissue, stabilizing nerve cells to prevent excessive firing, and calming nearby immune cells to prevent the release of substances that promote inflammation. The system can be seen as a bridge between body and mind. An understanding of this system might illuminate a mechanism that explains how states of consciousness can promote health or disease.

What Could Possibly Go Wrong?

Stimulating CB1 receptors promotes appetite. One implication of this response is that blocking or inhibiting the same receptor should lessen appetite. Sensing enormous potential profits, Big Pharma launched major research programs looking for an effective CB1 blocker. The Swiss drug company Sanofi-Aventis discovered, developed, and patented a selective CB1 receptor blocker named initially Acomplia, but later Rimonabant. Rimonabant very effectively binds to CB1 receptors. Because it binds to the receptor in a different way than endocannabinoids, the ECS system cannot activate the receptor naturally. In other words, the drug completely blocks the activation of the receptor (Barth and Rinaldi-Carmona 1999).

Blocking the ability of the ECS to activate CB1 receptors (and thereby contribute to hunger) made a lot of sense on paper. Animal trials used obese mice to test whether Rimonabant was effective at decreasing body weight. It was. Clinical trials soon started afterward, and the results looked promising—at least when the clinical endpoint was decreased weight. As it turns out, Rimonabant was also causing anxiety, depression, and suicidal thoughts in their subjects. It was identified as the cause of at least five deaths in the U.K. (Sam, Salem, and Ghatei 2011).

Rimonabant was classified as an anorectic antiobesity drug and was the first drug approved in that class. While never approved for use in the United States, it was approved in Europe in 2006 but withdrawn worldwide in 2008 due to the serious psychiatric side effects (Moreira and Crippa 2009).

The total number of endocannabinoid receptors in the body is believed to be greater than that of all other neuromodulator receptors combined, including receptors for serotonin and dopamine. Anandamide alone has the most receptors in the brain and is critical for maintaining a healthy central nervous system.

Because the ECS helps bring balance to the body, it is no surprise ECS changes have been observed in a number of diseases. Everything from neurodegenerative disorders to rheumatoid arthritis and cancer have shown changes in endocannabinoid levels, suggesting that the ECS may be an effective target for restoring balance in the body and promoting good health.

Cannabinoid receptors have been found in the sea squirt, an animal that evolved more than six hundred million years ago. Given its long evolutionary history, the endocannabinoid system must serve an important and basic function in animal physiology.

Phytohormones and Phytosteroids:
Ecology as Pharmacology

Yet another example of the complex and often confusing intersection of ecology, pharmacological medicine, and modern culture is the current focus on phytoestrogens. The word *hormone* is derived from Greek, meaning "set in motion." Hormones are chemicals secreted by both plants and animals to facilitate the regulation of physiological activities and maintenance of homeostasis. They are found in all multicellular organisms, and their role is to provide an internal communication system between cells located in distant parts of the body.

In animals, hormones are made by specialist cells, usually within an endocrine gland, and released into the bloodstream. They serve as chemical messengers and perform many roles at different targets. As a whole, the complex interplay between the glands, hormones, and target organs in animals is referred to as the endocrine system. Hormones affect many physiological activities, including growth, metabolism, appetite, puberty, and fertility.

In plants, hormones affect gene expression and transcription and influence the growth, development, and differentiation of cells and tissues. Unlike in animals, each plant cell is capable of producing hormones. The main plant hormones include abscisic acid, auxins, cytokinins, gibberellins, jasmonates, salicylic acid, and strigolactones.

Salicylic acid is well known to herbalists; its presence in a plant serves as an indicator of potential anti-inflammatory activity. Among its array of vital roles, salicylic acid is readily converted to methyl salicylate, a volatile molecule that has been shown to act as a long-distance signal to neighboring plants to warn of pathogen attack.

Jasmonate and its derivatives regulate a wide range of processes in plants. In particular, they are critical for plant defense and responses to poor environmental conditions. Although very widely found, they were first discovered in jasmine oils; hence the name. Some jasmonates are released as biogenic volatile organic compounds (BVOCs) to permit communication between plants in anticipation of mutual dangers.

As discussed in chapter 5, strigolactones are pivotal in the rich and complex ecology of plants interacting with the plethora of soil organisms. This involves physical contact between soil organism and plant, via the rhizosphere, where signal molecules mediate the different plant hormonal signaling pathways, leading to modifications in plant development and defense.

Signal molecules are an important feature of interactions between plants and free-living soil organisms. The same pathways are activated by different kinds of animals in the soil, such as bacteria, nematodes, and earthworms, with common consequences on plant growth, development, and defense. Plant hormonal activity is central to the multiple interactions that plants entertain with the community of soil organisms.

Human Hormones in Plants

Some plants make compounds that are usually thought of as human hormones. A study of 128 species from more than fifty plant families found progesterone in more than 80 percent, androgens in 70 percent, and estrogens in 50 percent. Estradiol and estrone have been detected in the seeds or pollen of apples, date palms, plums, and pomegranates, as well as quaking aspen catkins. Similarly, progestins are found in loblolly pine, common foxglove, tobacco, and elecampane. The leaves and flowers of chaste trees contain both progesterone and testosterone. Androstenedione is found in tobacco and elecampane. In aspen, estradiol content is correlated with flower maturation, suggesting that this hormone has important functions in the reproductive cycle of plants as well as animals.

However, a number of plant constituents that are not animal hormone analogues can be hormonally active. Known as phytosteroids, they are secondary metabolites found in plants that bind to hormonal steroid receptors in animals, including humans. They have a wide range of structures, sometimes quite different from those of human steroids, yet they can act as agonists or antagonists or, frequently, have mixed activity for many steroid receptors. Phytoestrogens are perhaps the best known, but there are other phytosteroids that bind to, for example, progesterone, androgen, and corticoid receptors.

Phytoestrogens mimic the activity of estrogens, a group of sex hormones that promote the development and maintenance of female characteristics in the human body. Note that there is no hormone called estrogen; rather, there are hormones that possess estrogenic activity. The three major hormones in humans that have estrogenic activity are estrone, estradiol, and estriol. They play an essential role in the growth and development of female secondary sexual characteristics and the regulation of the menstrual cycle and reproductive system. Their actions are mediated by the estrogen receptor, a protein that binds to DNA and controls gene expression.

Estrogens are found in all vertebrates as well as some insects. The existence of phytoestrogens that interact with animal hormone receptors suggests the possibility of a long coevolutionary history (Janeczko and Skoczowski 2005). With that in mind, any consideration of the therapeutic role of phytoestrogens necessitates an exploration of a fascinating nexus of issues, the complexity of which characterizes herbalism in modern culture.

Crossing Taxonomic Boundaries

Interest in hormonally active plants started in the 1940s and early 1950s, with the observation that some pastures abundant with species of clover had adverse effects on grazing sheep, causing "clover disease," where fertility dropped by 60 to 80 percent. It was found that this disease resulted from the consumption of phytoestrogens naturally present in this clover.

The resulting concern about the potential toxicity of phytoestrogens has led to two opposing perspectives: first, that they provide health benefits, and second, that they act as endocrine disruptors and threaten reproductive health.

Both points of view may be missing a key insight. These plant secondary metabolites communicate meaningfully across taxonomic boundaries. Consider, for example, the isoflavone genistein. In plants, it is involved in plant-bacteria communication; it recruits nitrogen-fixing bacteria to legume roots. In vertebrates, it can activate estrogen receptors that modulate reproduction, behavior, and metabolism. In amphibians and rodents, it alters thyroid hormone signaling. It is remarkable that one molecule can influence physiological function in plants and animals through such diverse mechanisms with a variety of outcomes (Tuli et al. 2019).

Fennel and Estragole, and the Breastfeeding Mother

Recently, concerns have been expressed about the potential carcinogenicity of constituents of fennel seed. The issues raised are a microcosm of the various concerns that appear at the interface of traditional herbal medicine with the scientific method. The constituents of concern are estragole and methyleugenol, present in the essential oil with a range of other constituents.

The potential carcinogenicity of estragole has led some governmental regulatory agencies to issue guidelines for the use of herbs that contain this constituent. For example, in 2002 the German Federal Institute for Health Protection of Consumers and Veterinary Medicine

(BgVV) advised that producers should reduce the content of estragole (and also methyleugenol) in foods as much as possible.

What are the issues concerning estragole and cancer? In mice, the liver metabolizes estragole to compounds that interact with DNA. This process is associated with an increased chance of genetic mutation and cancer. From this fact, it can be concluded that estragole has demonstrated carcinogenicity in mice and as such is a cancer hazard to mammals (Phillips et al. 1981; Drinkwater et al. 1976).

It is clear that estragole is a potential hazard (especially to mice), but this does not define the nature of the risk posed (if any) to humans. It is well known that different species have considerable differences in sensitivity to toxic chemicals. In particular, though both estragole and methyleugenol occur in humans, there are differences between how humans and rodents metabolize estragole.

When metabolized by the body, estragole produces toxic molecules, called epoxides, that can damage DNA by forming temporary bonds, called adducts, between strands. Crucially, such adducts are not found in humans because of efficient and rapid detoxification of estragole in the liver. No studies have reported any long-term health effects of human exposure to estragole. In fact, there is no human evidence pointing to a problem (Gori et al. 2012).

However, this is the point when things become convoluted! In *Medications and Mothers Milk 2017*, the seventeenth edition of one of the main texts on lactation pharmacology, the report on potential toxicity in the entry for fennel was changed from "moderately safe" to "possibly hazardous" (Hale and Rowe 2016). Nevertheless, fennel seeds have a long history as a pleasant and effective carminative and galactagogue. Many traditional herbal practices employ seeds from the Apiaceae family, such as fennel and anise, to promote lactation.

Can the Extrapolation Be Made from Mice to Humans?

Knowing that mice metabolize estragole differently than humans raises the question of whether dosages in mice have any relevance in humans. Even in rodents, studies show that signs of toxicity are minimal, probably in the dose range of one to ten milligrams per kilogram of mouse body weight, and that is approximately a hundred to a thousand times the anticipated human exposure to estragole. The daily exposure to estragole from food in people is in the range of 4.3 to 8.7 milligrams. Hager's Handbook, a standard German reference text, states that 100 milliliters of fennel tea, made from 6 grams of fennel seeds and 450 milliliters of water, contains only 0.4 milligram of estragole (Reuss 2013).

A more telling point is that estragole-containing plants are not a normal component of the diet of mice. In humans, exposure to estragole is well established and has developed over evolutionary time. The differences in metabolism suggests that humans have adjusted over the course of time to the naturally occurring amounts of estragole.

Single Constituents vs. Whole-Plant Profiles

The next issue is a common conceptual stumbling block. Can the properties of an herb be identified based on a single isolated constituent found in it? All the animal studies used purified estragole. In people, estragole enters the body as a component of fennel tea or in food that has been seasoned with an herb that contains it, such as fennel, basil, or tarragon. In other words, in the normal course of things, humans ingest estragole in the form of a complex phytochemical mixture.

If single-constituent data can be used as a basis for statements about an herb, then data about other constituents should also be considered. Fennel seed contains a whole range of antioxidant constituents, which might be considered protective against cancer genesis. Anethole, the main component of fennel essential oil, possess anti-inflammatory and anticarcinogenic actions. Thus, doubt remains that data from animal experiments can be extrapolated to humans (Parejo et al. 2002).

Consideration of these issues (dose, administration form, and differences in metabolism between species) raises doubts about the initial public conclusion that fennel seed can reasonably be anticipated to be a human carcinogen.

In 2023 the European Medicines Agency acknowledged that

extrapolating from research on estragole as a single constituent says little about complex herbal preparations that happen to contain estragole (EMA 2023). When researchers have studied whole-plant extracts that contain estragole, they have identified factors that interfere with many pharmacokinetic specifics, making dietary and herbal risk assessment for estragole problematic. The conclusion is that toxicity assessment for estragole-containing herbal medicinals seems not possible at the current time.

Science is revealing the pervasive presence of synergy in the ecology of the natural world and human organism. A fundamental role of plant secondary metabolites appears to be the facilitation of integration and homeostasis, promoting balance and health in the animals, including humans, that consume them. Indeed, as science continues to explore medicinal plants, the insights that flow from all the work done worldwide fundamentally support the idea of ecological holism. The great potential of herbs is not just as a window into how our world works, but as a contribution to human health and wholeness—and not only physical health but, from a systems biology perspective, also social and cultural health and well-being.

PART THREE

A Path Forward

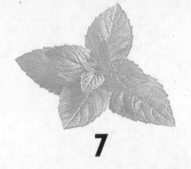

7

Herbalism Today

The logical next step in the conceptual progression explored in this book would be some affirmation of the growing cultural recognition of herbalism, the positive contribution it is making now, and its increasing relevance to the future.

Nevertheless, I cannot, in all faith, do that just yet—and not because I'm reacting to rapacious capitalist progress but because of a straightforward analysis of our current state of existence. Herbalism is now clearly present and playing a role in our culture, but in what reality?

The mere use of herbal medicines does not make a treatment holistic. Using an herbal tincture as a natural alternative to a prescription medication relegates the herb to the status of an organic drug delivery system. What makes herbs part of holistic treatment is the context within which the herbs are prescribed and used. It is important to recognize that, in and of itself, there is nothing unique or special about herbalism, but when approached from the appropriate perspective, it is uniquely relevant in very specific ways to the challenging years ahead. Herbalism is one aspect of the modern world in which ecological viability, not money and ownership, is the dominant issue. How humanity organizes itself and acts in the world will need to reflect such ecological realities. We can envision the generalities, but the specifics will be sure to surprise!

The triumphalism of neoliberal capitalism is an illusion based on wishful thinking. The reality of the global crisis has triggered a deep denial and subsequent rejection of personal, social, national, and cultural responsibility. The dominant culture's voracious brutalism has come face to face with ecological reality. It is being confronted by its past and present of destruction, greed, and human exceptionalism. The developed world is facing an existence vastly different from what it was promised. From the privileged crest of the breaking wave of three hundred years of capitalist delusion, the future must look intimidating. Wipeout indeed!

Putting the issue in the simplest and crudest way: There are far too many of us, and we have used up Earth's resources for what we considered important. Easy access to resources is over—no more industrial revolution, no more rare-earth-based smartphones, no more nonstick frying pans. In the twenty-first century's globalized economy, consumers are told that they can change the world by simply changing to a "green" brand, that humanity can consume its way out of overconsumption. This obvious lie is nothing more than a devious marketing ploy.

Although it has always been a part of human culture, herbalism has in recent years reappeared within Western societies, making itself visible in the modern world, manifesting in diverse and surprising ways. It finds itself playing many roles in fields from health care to the marketplace, personal empowerment, and cultural resilience.

Embracing herbalism can be one solid step out of the corporate miasma and a way of affirming life. But it so easily becomes a product line. The people's medicine has become a profit center. As much as the new science and data are proving insightful, they are also tools of the new empire. The herbal marketplace has become a way for corporate America to profit off herbalism, using slick greenwashing to convince the public that buying their goods will save them and/or the planet, and always with the aspiration to sell more and more. An opportunity to change our society's perspectives by re-valuing natural systems of ecology and homeostasis has degenerated into the gross pursuit of an ever-increasing bottom line.

Anything that points to positive change while still profiting in some way is dangerous misdirection based on the now unsupportable idea that growth is a social good. In the dominant culture, the way to suppress challenge is to buy it, so herbalists must beware of being subverted by the crumbs of cultural acceptance, the siren call of financial success, and the lure of mainstream respectability.

In its pure form, herbalism affirms and supports the resiliency of the human spirit—not the resilience of consumer society. It is a natural empowerment, grounded in the agency of ancient traditional ecological knowledge, that can help in the challenges of life in the Anthropocene.

Herbalism in the Marketplace

Herbalism in America finds itself in a cultural environment apparently created and maintained for the benefit of the marketplace. The rapidly growing herbal industry addressing the material needs of complementary medicine consumers is a manifestation of market forces—it is not a healing modality or a "holistic" anything, but an expression of the same rapacious economic forces that treat nature as a resource to control and profit from.

This system is obliterating cultural, biological, and herbal diversity. Embracing economics as the driving force for the field leads directly to standardization, not only in product development, but also in the development of treatment protocols. Regulators and manufacturers, who want to centralize, control, and standardize methods, ignore individual uniqueness (other than as a complicating factor). Practitioner knowledge and traditional wisdom are rarely acknowledged, so regulations, product lines, and research are predicated on abstract theories and piecemeal information.

Medicinal plants are clearly an important global resource in terms of health care, but they are also an important economic resource, traded extensively on scales ranging from the local to the international. Estimates of the size of the global herbal supplements market vary, but we can safely assume that it reached more than $30 billion in 2022. Much of that volume derives from stripping the natural world of its resources; only one-third of the herbs traded internationally are known to be in commercial cultivation (Jenkins, Timoshyna, and Cornthwaite 2018).

Within the world of international commerce and the regulations that control it, herbs are categorized as "medicinal and aromatic plants" (MAPs). MAPs are defined as botanical raw materials used for therapeutic, aromatic, and/or culinary purposes as components of cosmetics, medicinal products, health foods, and other natural health products. They are also the starting materials for value-added processed natural ingredients such as essential oils, dry and liquid extracts, and oleoresins. There is a growing demand for medicinal plants because of the increased production of herbal health care, cosmetic, dietary supplement, and medicinal products worldwide.

The growing use and trade of medicinal plants translates into traditional people's medicine being repurposed as a profit center. The growing presence of medicinal plants in the international marketplace means the commodification of herbs. The antidote? Resist commodification, build a sustainable supply chain, and understand regulation.

Resist Commodification

The term *commodification* describes the transformation of things into objects of trade. Our culture is brimming with things, whether goods, services, information, people, ideas, or even nature. Things can so easily become profits. This commodification has profoundly destructive implications for social life, with the pursuit of profit perverting human interactions, challenging the social contract, and corroding democracy. It is facilitated by what has been called financialization, a process in which the increasing importance of financial markets, institutions, and elites leads to an ever-growing influence on everything from national politics to daily life. The financialization of nature will only lead to the further commodification of social life (Davis and Kim 2015).

The all-encompassing nature of the polycrisis and inevitable planetary response of global environmental change will solve this profit- and greed-driven debasement of meaning. The underpinning of the global market's geocide will have the carpet pulled from under it. Ecological limits present the biggest threat to commodification and are a built-in solution delineated by the biosphere (Hermann 2021).

Build a Sustainable Supply Chain

It seems as though everyone involved in herbalism feels the need to heal and change the world, and of course this shows itself in many different ways, ways as diverse as the herbalists themselves. This is taking interesting forms at the interface of herbalism and international commerce. Supplying the needs of consumers confronts herbalism with all the issues of rapacious capitalism. On the spectrum of specifics, concerns about sustainability are paramount.

The more forward-thinking parts of the herb industry are attempting to address issues of sourcing and the supply chain more generally, within the context of sustainability. One example is the Sustainable Herbs Program (SHP), the focus of which is the supply chain and all its convolutions. This program is working to ensure that the vision and values of herbal medicine apply to the entire medicinal plant supply chain, aiming to show how changing this particular industry is a way to change the world.

A unique aspect of the SHP is its commitment to the market and work to make the supply chain more responsive to the challenges confronting it due to the climate crisis. The industry hinges on raw materials from Earth to fulfill consumer demand, creating a unique responsibility to regenerate and sustain those resources. This includes developing ways of doing business that regenerate the living systems on which those businesses depend.

What makes the SHP a refreshingly unique presence at the interface of herbalism, industry, and capitalism is the program's recognition of the paramount need of embracing holism, of seeing the whole ecosystem, human and nonhuman, as the basis for decisions made and actions taken. Rather than simply asking what's best for profitability, they encourage the industry to ask what is best for the plants and their ecosystems, as well as what is best for the communities whose liveli-hoods depend on those plants.

Traditional Medicinals

Traditional Medicinals (TM) is one of the most successful enterprises in the U.S. herb industry, with its products being pivotal in the development of organic pharmaceutical-quality herb teas. In 2004, I began working for TM as formulator and principal scientist. From its foundation in 1974, TM has been committed to social good and is one of the best examples of a commercially successful company working toward a better future, seeing the value in capitalism as a force for positive change.

Many of TM's products depend on imported herbs, leading the company to be an advocate for social and ecological sustainability. In cooperation with its supplier communities, TM initiatives include building schools, training health workers, improving water and food security, and providing women with opportunities for empowerment, all while preserving ancestral herbal knowledge. Consider, as examples, TM's work in the deserts of India, the grasslands of Paraguay, the steppes of Kazakhstan, and the panda forests of China.

Senna from the Desert

America has a high demand for laxatives. A common component of both over-the-counter and dietary supplement laxatives is senna, an herb native to the desert of Rajasthan, India. This is one of the hottest, driest places on Earth, where heat and scarcity of water are a constant challenge. Senna is drought-tolerant, but humans are not, leading TM to financially support and empower the communities that collect and cultivate senna for the company through the Revive! Project. Working with local communities, the project has facilitated programs that empower local leadership, as well as constructing rain water collection and storage systems, establishing community gardens, setting up cooperative banking, building schools, and awarding bicycle scholarships to improve access to distant secondary schools. TM views the project as an investment in its supplier communities, as a forward-thinking social business strategy, and as a manifestation of the principle that the only way a business can prosper is when all the parties involved prosper.

. . . .

Honey and Herbs in Paraguay

Paraguay is the source of citrus peel used in TM herbal teas. However, citrus farmers and wild collectors here face many financial challenges. Beekeeping is a common way to augment income in the Pampas region of Paraguay but often involves the challenging process of wild collection. To develop and stabilize this non-herbal income stream for its local citrus providers, TM offered beehives, along with technical training, to more than a hundred families in the region.

. . . .

Responsibly Sourced Licorice

Licorice root has been used in traditional Chinese medicine and ayurveda for more than five thousand years. Western medicinal use transcends licorice candies! In dietary supplements, licorice is used to soothe digestion and throat irritations, making wild-collected licorice from the steppes of Asia an important ingredient for TM. The company supports the well-being of collector communities by voluntarily paying above-market prices, helping to create economic stability with fair pay and steady employment.

Managing sustainable wild licorice populations involves harvesting half of the roots in a given area without returning for six years to allow enough time for regeneration of all species in the ecosystem and for roots to again reach maturity. Obviously, this cycle needs care and attention. In Kazakhstan, licorice grows abundantly but remotely, and to access it, collectors travel vast distances on bad roads, camping in the wilderness. With financing from TM the collectors voted to improve their camps with housing, clean water, electricity, and health care.

. . . .

Schisandra and Pandas

Some TM teas use wild-collected schisandra berries from China. Ethical collection is challenging, and commercialization is as much a social issue as an environmental one. The vines wind their way up and around host trees, with red berries growing in clusters, conventionally harvested by pulling down the vine and indiscriminately stripping off the berries. The sustainable practice TM harvesters use involves climbing the tree and carefully cropping the clusters of berries. Only the lower two-thirds of the vine is cropped, leaving the top third for wildlife to eat, and this way enabling seed dispersal and healthy plant regeneration. This skilled, time-consuming method makes sustainably harvested berries very expensive compared to the conventional crop. The vines grow in forests where endangered pandas live, so great care is needed to not only ensure herb quality but also minimize damage to the panda habitat.

Understand Regulation

The 1994 Dietary Supplement Health and Education Act (DSHEA) is usually perceived as having had a generally positive impact in the United States. But that is largely because of its success in making herbalism safe for capitalism, establishing a legal framework for the commodification of herbs and herbal products. The pros and cons of the DSHEA can be debated endlessly, but an unanticipated consequence has been the unintentional suppression of traditional insights and the insertion of market forces into yet another realm of healing.

When reading legislation, the most comprehensible section for non-lawyers often appears at the beginning of a bill under the heading "Findings." Here is found a rationale for the legislation, setting out Congress's intent and purposes. Notably, it is drafted in plain language by political congressional staff rather than technical drafters. The following material, from the DSHEA's findings, emphasizes the importance of information concerning dietary supplements.

(7) there is a growing need for emphasis on the dissemination of information linking nutrition and long-term good health; . . .

(13) although the Federal Government should take swift action

against products that are unsafe or adulterated, the Federal Government should not take any actions to impose unreasonable regulatory barriers limiting or slowing the flow of safe products and accurate information to consumers.

The DSHEA regulates the manufacture, safety, and marketing of dietary supplements, defining "dietary supplement" to mean a product (other than tobacco) intended to supplement the diet with a vitamin, a mineral, an herb or other botanical, or an amino acid. Such products must be labeled as dietary supplements and be intended for ingestion and must not be represented for use as conventional food or as a sole item of a meal or of the diet.

In the United States, it is against federal regulations to claim that these products prevent or treat disease. Companies are allowed to use what is referred to as "structure/function" wording if there is substantiation of scientific evidence for a supplement providing a potential health effect. Regulators do not require this substantiation to be at the level of significant scientific agreement that is required of drug claims. For dietary supplements, substantiation needs to be just "competent and scientific." Substantiation of this type is based on the informed professional opinion of some credentialed person, but it also acknowledges that information and experience from traditional knowledge and clinical experience have a role to play.

This sounds fair and balanced, but the end result is subjective. As it stands, the current regulatory structure strips herbal products of both their traditional context and their scientific documentation, leaving producers with a tidy marketplace but no room for consumers to engage with herbs in their traditional ecological matrix or scientific assessment. For herbalism to regain its independence from the grip of capitalism, regulations must be reworked so that claims based on historical or traditional use are either substantiated by scientific evidence or presented in such a way that consumers understand that the sole basis for the claim is a history of use of the product for a particular purpose.

Monographs Changing Tradition

An herb monograph is a detailed accounting of information about the herb, including a specification of its attributes and tests used to determine its quality. Authoritative monographs published in government pharmacopoeias have become central in research and manufacture, as the identity, quality, and purity standards contained in such monographs are critical to ensure the quality and safety of herbal medicines.

However, the inherent biases in evidence-driven medicine are leading to changes in this tradition—and as we shall see below, in the example of red clover, they are unfortunate. Compounding the problem, these changes are manifesting a general trend of dumbing down in otherwise very technically specific and accurate writing. The proliferation of "official" and "expert" materia medicas will prove a disservice, as paradoxically the more technically competent they appear, the more they tend to drop inconvenient bits of the herbal tradition that do not fit their paradigm of evidence-driven medicine, ignoring traditional uses and, instead, focusing exclusively on aspects of use that have been scientifically studied. The lack of evidence at the interface between modern medicine and traditional herbalism simply means no one got a grant!

For Example, Red Clover

A prime example concerns red clover (*Trifolium pratense*), long prized in European herbal medicine but relatively new to the mainstream and official pharmacopoeias. The range of indications for red clover that were recognized by herbalists included symptomatic alleviation of asthma and coughs and dermatological conditions such as eczema and psoriasis. Both topical and internal prescriptions were well-known. An important point is that the blossoms were the part of the red clover plant that was used, meaning that the historically accrued experience with this plant concerns the blossom, not the leaves.

In the 1990s, red clover leaves were found to be a relatively rich source of phytoestrogenic isoflavonoids that could be easily commercialized. The need for quality standards led to several official monographs being published. However, the focus of these monographs was on the leaves and levels of isoflavone present. This led to the development of red clover with relatively high levels of isoflavones in the leaves. No attention was given to maintaining, or even researching, the dermatological properties. The end result can be described as red clover as a drug delivery system for phytoestrogenic isoflavones. Traditional therapeutics were ignored in favor of the development of a commercial dietary supplement.

Therapeutic criteria for the various uses of red clover are covered in some excellent reviews for clinicians that can be found in the peer-reviewed literature (Nelsen et al. 2002) as well as in volume 4 of the five-volume World Health Organization Selected Medicinal Plants (WHO 2006).

The gaps in knowledge caused by such "evidence-driven" modernization will need to be compensated for by herbalists, medicine makers, and wildcrafters, or by those physicians, nurses, and pharmacists who are also accomplished herbalists and can bridge tradition with clinical science, hopefully clarifying the therapeutics of red clover.

An Exception:
The American Herbal Pharmacopoeia

Thankfully, there are exceptions to this trend around the world where the mainstreaming of traditional medicine is being chaperoned by knowledgeable, experienced herbalists. In the United States, this is epitomized by the American Herbal Pharmacopoeia (AHP), a non-profit educational organization that develops high-quality monographs on the herbs that are most frequently used in the United States. Each monograph provides information on botanical identification, chromatographic fingerprinting, cultivation, harvest, storage, potential adulterations, safety data, and appropriate sourcing, among other details. Most critical is the presence of competent therapeutic information that embraces multicultural traditional medicinal insights, with both historical and modern uses.

Of particular help to herbalists entering the market with their products, the AHP provides guidance on appropriate structure and function claims, dosages, interactions, side effects, contraindications, toxicology, and more. This information is critical for the development of substantiation files on structure and function claims, as required by the U.S. Food and Drug Administration.

Geo-authenticity versus Daodi

A subtle example of the cross-cultural confusion that intellectual appropriation causes concerns the Chinese concept of daodi and its interpretation in the West as geo-authenticity. Daodi is central to the use of medicinal plants in traditional Chinese medicine's holistic perspectives. Unfortunately, when these concepts are reinterpreted through Western lenses of sustainability and supply chain economics, it provides a window of opportunity for capitalists and governments to profit, regulate, and tax while looking like environmentalists.

Daodi, a concept unique to traditional Chinese medicine (TCM), is a way of identifying the quality of a medicinal material, while emphasizing therapeutic outcomes. Daodi has been interpreted in the West as being analogous to the French concept of terroir, the factors such as soil, climate, and sunlight that give wine grapes their distinctive character. Indeed, as one definition states, "Daodi medicinal material is produced and assembled in specific geographic regions with designated natural conditions and ecological environment, with particular attention to cultivation technique, harvesting, and processing" (Zhao, Guo, and Brand 2012). However, daodi is intricately related to clinical efficacy as well as macroscopic qualities such as taste and appearance. According to this concept, herb quality involves a matrix of factors ranging from clinical insight to geography, ecology, and horticulture. To these factors must be added the often unique traditional methods of preparation. The totality of these factors generates clinical outcomes that surpass products of the same herbs from other regions.

As the essence of Chinese medicinal materials, daodi has been playing an important role in health care for thousands of years. This accumulated clinical experience with medicinal substances has led to high-quality medicinal varieties being developed. There would be no concept of "daodi medicinal material" without this clinical experience. The whole concept of daodi and its application in practice is rooted in the documented history of TCM clinical practice. Among the five hundred or so commonly used Chinese medicinal materials, about two hundred have daodi specifications, accounting for 80 percent of the TCM medicinals in China.

Economic Drivers

Occasionally herbs from outside China have gained enough evidence of clinical efficacy in the TCM system that they have attained daodi status. Saffron, for example, cultivated in the West, was imported into China via Tibet. Known as xi hong hua, it became incorporated into the TCM materia medica and is valued for a range of properties. It is extremely expensive, needing around 160,000 flowers to produce a kilogram of saffron. However, it is now cultivated and prepared in China to daodi standards.

In 1702, a French priest described the use of Chinese ginseng (*Panax ginseng*) in Manchuria. This led to the discovery of American ginseng (*Panax quinquefolius*) near Montreal in 1716 (Persons 1994, 20). American ginseng from Canada was brought to China and became a valued item in the imperial court. Nowadays, American ginseng is successfully cultivated in China on a large scale and has achieved daodi status. Similarly, China now cultivates and uses maca root, an important food crop and medicinal plant native to Peru. This globalizing of herb cultivation occurs in all directions, with American cultivation of plants used traditionally in ayurveda and in TCM.

Daodi-quality medicines have become important items in international trade. In 2019, the total volume of TCM commodity imports and exports in China reached $6.174 billion, with the TCM industry becoming a key driver of development of China's health economy (Xiang et al. 2022). The promotion of TCM, and especially traditional medicines, is an important part of China's Belt and Road Initiative

(BRI), a global development strategy adopted by the Chinese government in 2013 to invest in 149 countries and international organizations. Worldwide trade in TCM services, including clinic treatment, education and training, and health tourism, is estimated to be at about $50 billion.

Globally, this is likely to increase both the demand for TCM and the sourcing of wild-sourced TCM ingredients from new areas. Any rapid increase in demand for wild resources risks exacerbating illegal and unsustainable trade, but with careful management, BRI and TCM could also present opportunities for well-governed supply chains, creating sustainable livelihoods for rural harvesters (Hinsley et al. 2020).

It appears that clinical components and traditional therapeutic insights are being dropped as China embraces the economic opportunities.

Geo-authenticity in the West

As we have seen, the context within which herbal quality is assessed and maintained is characterized by a profoundly holistic relationship. Therapists' clinical observation and experience, a raft of eco-physiological and geographic considerations, and the art and science of TCM medicine are all intimately involved in assessing daodi qualities. This highlights the difficulty of applying the principles in play without a major clinical component.

Recognizing the holistic relationship inherent in daodi highlights the fundamental difference between it and terroir. The quality of TCM medicines embraces factors from genetics to soil, geomorphology, and pharmaceutical specifics. Most especially, and impressively, patient outcome and clinical observation are central to the concept of quality. Quantifiable levels of specific constituents, region of origin, and harvesting and handling issues, while crucial, have to be seen in the context of how real people respond therapeutically. Terroir of wine just identifies the quality and source of the inebriation!

The European Commission adopted a geographical indications system for wines, spirit drinks, and agricultural products. This system could potentially include herbs. The measures are intended to benefit the rural economy and achieve a higher level of protection for the agricultural sector. The intention is to maintain the EU's high food quality and standards, ensuring the preservation of cultural, gastronomic, and local heritage. For the commission, this means regulations that certify authenticity within the EU and across the world.

In 2007, the World Intellectual Property Organization organized a conference on the use of geographical indications for agricultural products and foodstuffs. They proposed the creation of a Protected Designation of Origin certification, which would circumscribe a region within which the product in question originated, meaning that it possesses characteristics that are essentially or exclusively due to that geographical environment (recognizing its inherent natural and human factors) and regional production, processing, and preparation methods.

This has, as an example, taken the form of chamomile from the Czech Republic being certified under this system, exclusively able to be marketed with designation of "Chamomilla Bohemica." This may be an excellent promotional marketing tool for that part of central Europe, but what is it saying about chamomile from anywhere else? Are the regulators saying that the chamomile grown in Wales, used by herbalists in clinical practice, is not authentic? The attempt to make the profoundly holistic concept of daodi a marketing tool in capitalism's commodification of herbalism is unfortunate, but very predictable.

Herbalism as Tulip Mania

The recent cultural infatuation with cannabidiol (CBD) is the epitome of herbalism as product—tulip mania resurfacing to engulf cannabis. Tulip mania was the first recorded speculative bubble, and the term is now a metaphor for any economic bubble in which prices stray too far from intrinsic values. It dates from the mid-1630s, when the newly affluent Dutch became enamored of tulips. After their introduction into Europe from Ottoman Turkey, tulips had rapidly become a coveted luxury item, and a profusion of varieties followed. Some of these tulips were vividly multicolored, with intricate lines and flame-like streaks. Bulbs that engendered such spectacular blooms became highly sought after—and valuable. According to contemporary reports, the tulip frenzy reached a point where some bulbs sold for what amounted to more than ten times the annual income of a skilled artisan (Mackay 1841).

(Side note: The variegated coloring of tulip blooms is actually due to infection by mosaic virus.)

Tulip mania exemplifies a core issue facing herbalism today: Commodification enables the ownership, profit, and greed that are characteristic of the dominant culture, leading to the disempowerment of the noncorporate. In turn, the cultural paradigm becomes centered around facilitating the workings of the marketplace, and very soon the "commons," the greater whole, becomes a barrier to trade and thus a cultural negative.

This leads to an all-pervasive capitalist miasma in our society. The fog is so omnipresent and unavoidable that we have been educated and conditioned into internalizing the capitalist agenda. The very fact of the primacy of the herb "industry" in the herb "world" illuminates this state. There is no specific conspiracy involved, just very successful thought control, the same manipulation everyone in the culture is being exploited by.

Capitalism is a system of using of money to make money, not to make a living. Buying and selling are *commerce*, not capitalism, and yet in the current era, capitalism has infiltrated and commandeered all commercial endeavors, pushing profit into primacy over people. The banks, stock markets, and speculators of the world are a profoundly negative force, transforming commerce into capitalism globally, locally, and, most specifically for our purposes, in herbalism.

In this capitalist distortion we live in, we can resist the commoditizers by denying "the divine right of capital" (Kelly 2001). A fundamental challenge of the capitalist worldview is that it holds nature as something to conquer, commercialize, and profit from, rather than recognizing that *we* are nature. Resisting commodification would mean seeing herbs not as potential new drugs, alternative medicine, or dietary supplements, but as a core aspect of life on this planet—nature as us, not a thing to be conquered.

The dominant culture's embrace of herbalism is not necessarily something to affirm. I am affirming the fundamental nature of the RESISTance: a timeless expression of the green in the face of humanity's environmental pillaging.

Woke Herbalism

The complexity of the issues facing herbalism in the twenty-first century needs herbalists to be thoughtful, aware, and attentive to the plethora of nonherbal (yet still important!) concerns. The burgeoning response to climate change being expressed by all aspects of the herbal world is a wonderful thing, a vehicle for people's heartfelt response to heal everything from humans to the biosphere, from the soil to supply chains. However, there is a lot more to consider. In other words, herbalism needs to be woke! Recognizing and combating racial prejudice, discrimination, economic and cultural oppression, and especially the repercussions of the slave trade and Eurocentrism are paramount. We'll explore some of the implications below.

Imperial Roots and Ravages

The modern herb industry, and the herbalism it caters to, has its roots in the slave trade and colonialism. This reality needs acknowledgment in order to enable recognition of the insidious distortions it has bequeathed to both herbalism and the marketplace.

Ships visiting Africa and the Americas were private vessels engaged in the "triangular trade." That three-way exchange sent guns and manufactured goods to Africa, enslaved people to the Americas, and dyes, drugs, and sugar back to Europe. Of course, the "drugs" were medicinal plants.

Among the multitude of obscenities that characterized the slave trade was the destruction of the pristine forest of what became Carolina.

The British empire was built on the strength of its navy, which consisted entirely of wooden ships. In other words, entirely of dead forests. Perhaps the most famous is HMS *Victory*, Lord Nelson's flagship at the Battle of Trafalgar in 1805. According to records, the *Victory* was constructed from approximately six thousand trees, or about a hundred acres of woodland, 90 percent of which was oak, but also elm, fir, pine, and spruce. The tree of life (*Guaiacum* spp.) was also used in small quantities. The thickness of the hull at the water line was approximately two feet.

By the seventeenth century, Britain's forests were almost denuded of the old-growth oak trees essential for the warships demanded by imperialism and the growth of empire. However, the New World colonies solved this supply problem with a longleaf pine (*Pinus palustris*) forest that extended over ninety million acres, including North Carolina's coastal plain and much of the southern Piedmont. The abundance of pine trees and their use as timber and especially naval stores was crucial in the North Carolina colony's economy. Originally, "naval stores" referred to everything used to build a ship, including wood and cloth, but the term gradually came to mean just tar, pitch, and turpentine. All were manufactured from pine trees, turpentine being distilled from a gum that the trees secrete to protect wounds in their trunks. The high demand decimated the longleaf forest. Today, even centuries after the era of wooden ships, the longleaf pine has nearly vanished from the landscape, reducing the ecosystem to 5 percent of its original range (USDA 2024).

The longleaf pine has some unique ecological features. It is specially adapted to forest fires. Its seeds germinate and put down roots rapidly in the bare mineral-rich soil following a fire. Seedlings stay low to the ground to survive further fire, then undergo a growth spurt that puts their fire-sensitive needles above the flames. Mature trees have fire-resistant bark. Because most trees are quickly killed by fire, the longleaf was the only tree thriving in its forests, with great spaces between mature trees. In those open spaces, grasses and specially adapted flowers grow. The result is a unique and irreplaceable ecosystem, once called the "longleaf pine savanna" because it was a kind of grassland of trees.

Its loss is just another footnote from the annals of the empire. Was it worth it?

Terminology of Oppression

Euro-American scientific tradition carries the burdens of historic colonialism and barriers to participation for those who come from outside Europe and the United States. To see an example, simply look to the sky. Hundreds of species of birds across South America, Central Africa, China, and the Pacific Islands were named by American and European scientists during periods of colonial control. Only recently have movements such as #BirdNamesForBirds emerged to restore Indigenous descriptive names.

The study of linguistic relativism has shown that the way people think of the world is influenced directly by the language they use to talk about it. The conditioning of patriarchal imperialism and its all-encompassing yet insidious worldview can be seen in the way science names the living world. This is meant not as a challenge to the content and work of taxonomy, but as a semantic concern about taxonomy's impact on viewpoint.

The highest grouping used in taxonomic ranking is the domain or empire. There are three domains, the Archaea, Bacteria, and Eukarya, recognizing fundamental biological differences. Just below domain is the rank of kingdom, which in turn is divided into smaller groups called phyla. The United States and Canada use a system of six kingdoms (Animalia, Plantae, Fungi, Protista, Archaea, and Bacteria), while Europe and much of the rest of the world use five (Animalia, Plantae, Fungi, Protista, and Monera). When this system was introduced in the eighteenth century, the highest rank was kingdom, followed by class, order, genus, and species. Eventually two more ranks were introduced, making the sequence kingdom, phylum, class, order, family, genus, and species. The rank of domain was introduced above kingdom in 1990. All of which has been a boon to biology in ways too numerous to list.

However, if the nonbiological definitions of these words are considered, things become very political, very quickly. A murky miasma of imperialism starts to rise from the still waters of scientific objectivity. This culturally loaded language needs deconstructing, but there is no need for careful semantic analyses to expose any hidden internal assumptions and contradictions. A simple dictionary search reveals everything!

The various definitions of *domain* refer to territory owned or controlled by a ruler or government. In the field of information technology, a domain is a network of computers and devices that are controlled by one authority with specific guidelines. More specifically, a domain is controlled by one particular company that has its own internet presence and IP address. The emphasis is on central singular control.

One synonym for *domain* is *empire*, defined as an aggregate of many separate states or territories under a single supreme authority, especially an emperor or empress. In other words, the central organizing structure of taxonomy is a reflection of European monarchy, all power and control flowing from a central figure with hierarchical control of all within its domain.

The next nested taxonomic ranking is kingdom. Leaving out the biological meaning of kingdom, Webster's dictionary gives a number of definitions. The main entry involves the political kingdom, an organized community or major territorial unit having a monarchical form of government headed by a king or queen. The second definition refers to the eternal kingship of God, in the Christian sense. The third meaning is a realm or region in which something is dominant or an area or sphere in which one holds a preeminent position. Again, we see in this categorization the hierarchical flow of power from the center to the periphery.

Fascist Forces: Nazi Botany

History shows that an environmental, green, or herbal orientation is not inherently a social good. A strange synthesis of plants and politics occurred in 1930s Germany, when botany become nationalism and herbalism became fascist. The horror of the Nazi regime has been well documented—the definition of "crimes against humanity" was created to describe what they did—but, for our purposes, we will look at a rarely acknowledged herbal example that is relevant here.

The Nazis applied their antagonism toward anything non-German to native plants and herbs, attempting to eliminate foreign plants from Germany. The idea was "to cleanse the German landscape of unharmonious foreign substance" (Wolschke-Bulmahn 1995). The "fight" against foreign plants was compared with the fight of the Aryan nation against all others.

As an example of the insanity such fascist ideas leads to, consider impatiens. Impatiens is a genus (*Impatiens* spp.) of more than a thousand species of flowering plants, widely distributed throughout the Northern Hemisphere. Nazi botanists proposed a "war of extermination" against the species *Impatiens parviflora*, categorizing it as a stranger that dared to spread and compete with *I. nolitangere*, a similar species considered native to Germany. "As with the fight against Bolshevism," a team of German botanists proclaimed in 1942, "our entire Occidental culture is at stake, so with the fight against this Mongolian invader, an essential element of this culture, namely, the beauty of our home forest is at stake" (Groening and Wolschke-Bulmahn 1992).

Although the Nazi regime considered plants native to Germany to be superior to plants from outside Germany, there was no definition of what constituted a German plant. In practice, plants became "German" through years of association with German people. This meant many non-native food crops and herbs were likely considered native by Nazi officials and scientists, including potatoes, which originated in South America but were popular in Germany, and sweet cherries (*Prunus avium*), which evolved in Asia Minor but were widely cultivated in Germany.

Nazi fascination with all things "natural" extended to native herbs, herbalism, and homeopathic medicine (Otto 1993). Several large research projects were started to test which natural soil treatments (amendments) produced the best results. Some of these experiments were conducted in concentration camps, where the worst violations of ethical standards in the history of medicine occurred under the direct supervision and responsibility of German doctors. The Dachau concentration camp was the site of a 510-acre plantation of medicinal plants with greenhouses, herb drying and processing facilities, and a research institute exploring a range of herbal issues. The workers were all slave laborers from the concentration camp, most of whom died. The plantation was created under the auspices of Heinrich Himmler, a main architect of the Holocaust, who directed the murder of millions of people.

This is not simply an unpleasant part of the tapestry of herbal history, but a reminder that fascism can arise anywhere at any time—who would have expected it to be a major force in twenty-first-century U.S. politics?

Having looked at some of the forces feeding these shadows in our society and even within herbalism itself, there is an obvious need for reconciliation as part of humanity's healing process, acknowledging oppression in all its overt and deviously subtle manifestations. Herbalism is a modality that is uniquely suited to the healing of the oppressed, contributing in various ways to the restoration of health. This might be the alleviation of the distress of illness through healing the physical body or the more profound work of healing the split between humanity and nature. While one is based on individual responses to therapeutic herbs and the other is a transformation of consciousness, both are expressions of herbs at work. The simple gifts bestowed by these plants can play a transformative role at many levels of our lives, whether considering individuals, communities, or nations.

Herbalism, in the context of holistic medicine, recognizes and affirms the uniqueness of each individual. In other words, from an herbalist's perspective, diversity and variation are normal, and a worldview that seeds such natural diversity in a negative light is itself an abomination. Herbalism affirms people, not the organizations and laws devised by the dominant culture to control the "other." It affirms nature and ecology as an organizing principle, recognizing all our relatives (human, animal, and plant) as having undeniable rights and the planet as our shared home. It is a healing modality that by its very nature supports the choice to live in a decentralized way, decolonizing the mind by freeing oneself from old imperialist, capitalist, and/or fascist conditioning and embracing lifestyles that value the small, the community, and integration with the natural world.

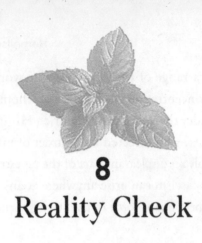

8
Reality Check

So let us not talk falsely now, the hour is getting late.
BOB DYLAN, "ALL ALONG THE WATCHTOWER"

Gaia and her perspectives are emerging in human consciousness. One of these timely manifestations is the surprising reappearance of herbalism within modern culture. From the multitarget pharmacology of flavonoids to the refugia of traditional herbal knowledge and more, herbalism has much to offer modernity. The upwelling of herbalism is one aspect of the collective consciousness's response to the hastening global environmental change and the concurrent withering of human spirit.

The planet-wide use of herbs—in our species' ancestors, in animals, and in all the cultures of modern humans—suggests that herbalism connects with something fundamental in our biology. Its omnipresence is a clear justification for exploring ecology, cellular biology, and pharmacology from an herbal perspective. As well, given that secondary metabolite profiles in plants are mediated by their environment, and given the biochemical intimacy of the relationship between secondary metabolites and human well-being that has been developing over deep time, the accelerating pace of planet-wide environmental changes should raise red flags.

A cultural map of herbalism in the United States of 2020 might have illuminated many aspects of its reappearance. However, this trend may not be as positive as you might think—not because of herbalism, but because of the culture! Herbalism finds itself at a nexus of many of the most challenging issues of our time: to cite a few, globalization, runaway capitalism, extreme inequalities, planetary environmental change, and the very real possibility of ecological collapse.

How can we name the world's ongoing crises when words like *disaster*, *catastrophe*, or *emergency* don't suffice? Experts have coined the term *polycrisis* to describe the potential for deeply interconnected systems to erode or collapse in tandem. On its website, the Canadian Cascade Institute defines a polycrisis as "any combination of three or more interacting systemic risks with the potential to cause a cascading, runaway failure of Earth's natural and social systems that irreversibly and catastrophically degrades humanity's prospects." The term is now used by international bodies from the United Nations to the World Economic Forum to describe the simultaneous, overlapping crises facing the world, where apparently unrelated shocks caused by different crises interact so that the whole is even more overwhelming than the sum of the parts.

It is not simply lots of crises but one polycrisis, characteristic of an interconnected, interdependent world. It is not just a new geological period, the Anthropocene, but a new phase of history, different from anything in the past. Population growth, technological change, the spread of global capitalism, and what has been called the Great Acceleration—the dramatic surge across a large range of measures of human activity—has pushed many ecological systems to their limits (Shoshitaishvili 2021). The overwhelming size and nature of this multifaceted crisis is the defining reality of the twenty-first century.

However, the mainstream response has ranged from denial to hand-wringing and another conference! Put into the context of the planetary polycrisis human culture itself has precipitated, the response can be seen as a death wish. The situation was perhaps put best by UN Secretary-General António Guterres, in a speech on September 10, 2018, demanding urgent action from world leaders (note the crucial, now-expired date of 2020):

> If we do not change course by 2020, we risk missing the point where we can avoid runaway climate change, with disastrous consequences for people and all the natural systems that sustain us. . . . Scientists have been telling us for decades. Over and over again. Far too many leaders have refused to listen. Far too few have acted with the vision the science demands.
>
> We know what is happening to our planet. We know what we need to do. And we even know how to do it. But sadly, the ambition of our action is nowhere near where it needs to be. . . . We have the moral and economic incentives to act. What is still missing . . . is the leadership, and the sense of urgency and true commitment to [a] decisive multilateral response. . . .
>
> Our fate is in our hands. The world is counting on all of us to rise to the challenge before it's too late.

Since the first UN environmental conference in Stockholm in 1972, there have been a plethora of proposals to mitigate the looming polycrisis. This is not the place to explore them, but the recognition that such a response is underway is crucial. Vast numbers of people around the world, and organizations they have formed, are committed to this endeavor.

Why is there no substantive political or economic response? The challenges posed by the global environmental change are not primarily technical in nature. Of course, a daunting array of profound problems face humanity, but they are addressable with technologies and resources that currently exist. These resources could be the basis for sustainably retooling technology and empowering people as they work toward a viable future. The issue is a lack of not knowledge, technology, or resources but intention.

Why No Response?

Perhaps personal cognitive biases contribute to humanity's seeming lack of will to act on climate change. For example, with the cognitive bias known as hyperbolic discounting, people see the present as more important than the future, which impedes their ability to see the prospect of complex challenges in the time ahead. Or they may lack concern for future generations, doubting whether sacrifices in the present in order to benefit future generations are worth it. Then there is the bystander effect, the presumption that someone else will deal with any crisis, assuming that leaders are doing something about climate change.

However, the lack of response to the ongoing polycrisis is not simply the result of individual psychology. It must be acknowledged that there have been active campaigns to manufacture doubt about the science behind climate change, obscuring the scientific consensus and data, questioning whether climate change is caused by humans, and downplaying its effects on nature and human society, all contributing to government inaction worldwide.

At the same time, the very real threat of climate change is causing an epidemic of eco-anxiety, which the American Psychology Association describes as "the chronic fear of environmental cataclysm that comes from observing the seemingly irrevocable impact of climate change and the associated concern for one's future and that of next generations."

A key factor in easing eco-anxiety is taking meaningful actions to gain a sense of agency and build personal resilience. In this way, the dark emotions evoked by the polycrisis can be the basis for empowerment and progress. A recent paper in the well-respected medical journal *The Lancet* put climate anxiety in context by saying it "may be the crucible through which humanity must pass to harness the energy and conviction that are needed for the lifesaving changes now required" (Cunsolo et al. 2020).

Fear is not simply something to be overcome but also a tool for mobilization. For activists, fear of the consequences of inaction is often a spur to action. In these days, fear, anger, and hope are the principal emotions that shape environmental action.

Global Catastrophic Risks
and Global Governance

The response of central governments and international finance institutions—in fact, the whole panoply of organizational response to the clearly existential threat—is pathetically inadequate and criminally myopic. Any objective analysis of the issues leads to a recognition of the need to act *now*.

A surprising voice of climate reason is the U.S. Department of Defense (DoD). The U.S. military not only acknowledges climate change but is actively preparing for its potential havoc. Since the release of its first report on climate change in 2015, the DoD has been at the forefront of meaningful and rational evaluation of climate concerns, from the increasing need for humanitarian assistance and disaster response capabilities to political tensions caused by the melting arctic ice and the demand for specialized cold-weather military equipment for U.S. forces. It also recognizes that supply chain resilience is an ever-growing problem, seeing the various ways climate change will impact production and shipping. DoD places what it calls "climate intelligence" at the center of informed decision-making. In other words, the department recognizes the importance of facts about the issues, not avoidance and denial of the challenging reality.

DoD and each department of the military have developed action plans. They've produced glossy brochures that read like rational, well-conceived approaches to the polycrisis. However, this is the military, a national killing machine. Any positive moves by the DoD to combat climate change must be seen as ways to maintain military dominance in the face of climate risks. For example, the 2022 Air Force Climate Action Plan is designed to ensure resilience to the effects of climate change in order to "sustain a combat-credible force and enable global power projection" (Department of the Air Force 2022).

In the absence of any united global response, a few governments, corporations, organizations, and people themselves are attempting to mitigate and prepare for global catastrophes. This people-based response is one of the few positive signs of recent years. However, there are forces opposing such mitigation endeavors. The resurgent far right is but one example, fomenting a deeply disturbing and toxic oppositional response that is reactionary in all senses of that word.

To clarify, *reactionary* is not synonymous with *conservative*. In common usage, *reactionary* describes a person or policy opposing progressive change or promoting return to a past social condition. The reactionary worldview favors a return to a previous political state believed to possess characteristics that are absent from the contemporary status quo. It is a point of view meant to restore a past status quo. It is fundamentally patriarchal in its worldview, seeing "human nature" as imprinted on humanity by evolution and/or God. Hierarchy is seen not as problematic but as desirable, and something not be challenged.

This might, possibly, be a valid political perspective from which to address politics, but *that is not the nature of the problem*. The problem is not human constructs, theories, or belief systems but planetary effects and outcomes that rise above politics and belief.

Reactionary critiques are often imbued with a longing for some past greatness or "golden age." However, there is no golden past to return to, no golden past of benevolent kings, no golden past of patriarchal justice. Concepts of the golden age come from the oppressors to justify the "greatness" that characterizes their oppression, and not from those they oppress. When the oppressed have no voice, the golden age is always a fascist illusion.

The Greek poet Hesiod first mentioned a "golden age" set in about 700 BCE, describing it as an age when all humans were created directly by the Olympian gods. They lived long lives in peace and harmony, oblivious of death. But this classical "golden age" was also a purely mythical creation—these humans of Olympian creation also had no women and so could not reproduce.

Later ideas of a historical golden age are generally cultural propaganda. For example, one of the Spanish golden ages is considered to be the Spanish empire between the sixteenth and seventeenth centuries. However, this was also the time of the Spanish Inquisition, so it was not all that golden if you were Jewish. The golden age of England is said to be the Elizabethan era, in the late sixteenth century, but not if you were Catholic. The Victorian era is often described as the golden age of Britain, and it may have been so unless you were a Welsh-speaking Welshman, a worker in what William Blake described as the "dark satanic mills," or a colonized African "subject."

In other words, the reactionary nature of the far right political agenda has no true footing in its desire to turn back the clock to a "golden age" of political, economic, and social vitality. No such thing exists, and in fact never did.

It is arguable that efforts to address the polycrisis through the centralized application of technology and blind trust in the vagaries of the marketplace are worsening all they touch. International attempts to "weather the storm" are essential, but if they are dependent on international capital and the reactionary forces they represent, the inherent contradictions will stymie even the best-intentioned and scientifically sound programs.

The Anthropocene Epoch

In the past 250 years, human-driven global change has caused climate change, widespread species extinctions, desertification, ocean acidification, ozone depletion, pollution, and other large-scale shifts. The changes have been so rapid and all-encompassing that a change in the geological epoch has been proposed. The climatic, biological, and geochemical signatures of human activity in sediments and ice cores suggests that the era since the mid-twentieth century should be recognized as a geological epoch distinct from the previous Holocene. The new Anthropocene epoch, as it's known, takes its name from a combination of *anthropo-*, "human," and *-cene*, "new" or "recent."

In the Earth sciences, the planet is considered in terms of different spheres. The geosphere includes all the rocks making up the crust, mantle, and core. The lithosphere is the part of the geosphere made up of surface rocks and landforms. The pedosphere is the soil. Planetary water, both salt and freshwater, is described as the hydrosphere. The frozen water of the ice caps and permafrost is the cryosphere. The atmosphere is Earth's envelope of gases, consisting of (from bottom to top) the troposphere, stratosphere, mesosphere, and thermosphere. All these spheres, together, provide the habitat for the biosphere, the global ecological system integrating all living beings and their relationships with each other and the environment, comprising the totality of biodiversity (Ellis and Haff 2009).

These spheres have been in existence, in one form or another, for most of the planet's 4.6 billion years of existence. However, the Anthropocene epoch appears to be creating new spheres, such as the technosphere, encompassing all of the technological objects manufactured by humans. It comprises not just machines but the professional and social systems through which people interact with technology. It also includes the agricultural technology use to facilitate the production of enormous numbers of animals for food, the vast acreage of crops cultivated to sustain both animals and humans, and the soils that are extensively modified from their natural state to carry out this task. It includes all the roads, railways, airports, mines, quarries, oil and gas fields, cities, and engineered riverways and reservoirs. This means the technosphere also includes the debris of their ends. Anthropocene civilization generates extraordinary amounts of waste, from landfill sites to pollution in the air, soil, and water.

Recent geological times have been named after plants, as in the Lesser Dryas period, dating from twelve thousand to fifteen thousand years ago, which is named after the mountain avens, *Dryas octopetala*. A sign of our times is naming deposits after the technology that created them. The digital age is replete in future technofossils. By definition, a fossil is biologically made, robust, and resistant to decay, which certainly characterizes the detritus of the technosphere. Just consider the fate of generations of handheld devices. Following ideas from paleontology, they may well be used as index fossils to characterize strata of the Anthropocene. Index fossils define and identify different geologic periods; they must have a short vertical range in strata (relatively short existence), wide geographic distribution, and rapid evolutionary trends.

This makes the robust mobile phone ideal, thanks to its worldwide usage and rapid design change. It is not known how many varieties of technofossils exist, as the number is continually increasing as technological evolution continues. These technofossils are found in new forms of rock, such as plastiglomerate, a rock made of a mixture of sedimentary grains and other natural debris (like shells or wood) that is held together by plastic.

The biosphere is extremely good at recycling the material it is made of, whereas the technosphere is appalling at it. Some of the waste is obvious, like the plastics accumulating in the world's oceans and shorelines. Other waste is not, being colorless and odorless, like carbon dioxide. It has been estimated that this mass—everything from old technology and concrete to Barbie dolls—currently totals thirty trillion tons, or nearly forty pounds per square foot on the surface of Earth. Today, this crust of our old stuff outweighs us by a ratio of sixty thousand to one (Duarte Santos 2021).

Obviously, this is extremely problematic, calling for drastic steps to address the sources of waste and the technosphere itself. However, in a perverse catch-22, the technosphere keeps populations alive through the food and other resources it provides. Its development has allowed the human population to grow from the few tens of millions that could be supported by hunter-gatherers to the eight billion of 2023. For example, just one technological innovation, artificial fertilizers, keeps about half the human population alive. Bear in mind that the United Nations expects the world's population to increase by nearly two billion persons over the next thirty years, rising to 9.7 billion in 2050 and possibly peaking at nearly 10.4 billion in the mid-2080s.

Of more importance than the details are the psychological and cultural complexities that underlie decision-making. The unquestioned preeminence given to technological development and to the drive for profit is very problematic. The existential threat posed by the polycrisis raises issues that transcend economics, as will be explored below. The ongoing mass species extinction and loss of biodiversity, directly caused by the drive for profit, will not be reversed by invoking devious new capitalist "green" programs that sell hope in service of enriching the elite.

Biodiversity Loss

Healthy communities rely on well-functioning ecosystems providing clean air, fresh water, medicines, and food. Well-functioning ecosystems also limit disease and stabilize the climate. As the ongoing pace of bio-diversity loss builds at an unprecedented rate, it degrades and disrupts ecosystems, so that they are no longer able to provide services (like fresh water, food, and fuel). The direct impact of these changes on human health is becoming evident worldwide. Indirectly, changes in ecosystem services affect livelihoods, income, and migration patterns and, on occasion, may even cause or exacerbate political conflict. Additionally, biological diversity of microorganisms, flora, and fauna provides extensive benefits for biological and pharmacological sciences. Significant medical and pharmacological discoveries are made through greater understanding of Earth's biodiversity. Loss in biodiversity may limit the discovery of potential treatments for many diseases and health problems.

To quantify biodiversity loss, the logical first step would be knowing how many species are on Earth currently. That would seem to be fundamental data, but the number remains uncertain, with estimates ranging from about two million species to approximately one trillion. Until recently most estimates pointed to around eleven million species, but new technology has found a previously unsuspected number of species of bacteria and viruses in the world's oceans. When this vast diversity of oceanic microbiology is added to counts, estimates suggest there are at least one to six billion species on Earth (Larsen et al. 2017). There is greater certainty about the decline in the number of species. Theory and findings suggest that species are dying off a thousand times more frequently now than before the arrival of humans sixty million years ago (De Vos et al. 2015).

The reduction in biodiversity that human domination has caused is reflected in the fact that livestock and humans far outweigh wild animals. Since the beginning of human civilization, 83 percent of mammals have disappeared. Today livestock make up 60 percent of the biomass of all mammals left, followed by humans at 36 percent, and with wild mammals being only 4 percent. In 2021, a total of 37,400 species were considered threatened with extinction, compared to 16,119 in 2006.

Much international work prioritizes conservation efforts, and many governments have conserved land under the Convention on Biological Diversity (CBD), a multilateral treaty signed in 1992. Since 2010, approximately 164 countries have developed plans to reach their conservation targets, including the protection of 17 percent of terrestrial and inland waters and 10 percent of coastal and marine areas. The emphasis here is on "developed plans." Unfortunately, much of the planning has not been put into practice.

When the Intergovernmental Science-Policy Platform on Biodiversity and Ecosystem Services (IPBES) published its Global Assessment Report on Biodiversity in 2019, the report stated that up to a million plant and animal species are facing extinction because of human activities. The 2020 United Nations Global Biodiversity Outlook report highlighted that if the status quo is not changed, biodiversity will continue to decline due to "currently unsustainable patterns of production and consumption, population growth and technological developments." This led sixty-four nations and the European Union to pledge to halt environmental degradation. But China, India, Russia, Brazil, and the United States were not among them.

Sir Peter Scott, founder of the World Wide Fund for Nature (better known in the United States as the World Wildlife Fund) and one of the best-known ornithologists in the U.K., clearly expressed the despondency felt: "You know, when we first set up WWF, our objective was to save endangered species from extinction. But we have failed completely; we haven't managed to save a single one. If only we had put all that money into condoms, we might have done some good" (Short 2010).

The geological record shows that Earth has experienced numerous mass extinction events, with five main ones. An event 443 million years ago caused the extinctions of 60 to 70 percent of all species. Then,

360 million years ago, 70 percent of species disappeared, including almost all corals. The largest mass extinction occurred 250 million years ago, during which 95 percent of all species perished; it was linked to massive volcanism in Siberia that caused extreme global warming. Another event 200 million years ago led to 75 percent of species dying off, leaving Earth clear for dinosaurs to flourish. Then, 65 million years ago, a giant asteroid impact in what is now Mexico saw the end of the dinosaurs and ammonites.

An interesting aside concerns a geologically recent smaller extinction event that took place during the Younger Dryas period approximately thirteen thousand years ago. This period, temporarily interrupting a longer climatic warming trend, saw a return to glacial conditions just before the warmer Holocene. In the geologic record, the rocks dated to the Younger Dryas period are characterized by the pollen of a plant found today, the beautiful alpine wildflower, *Dryas octopetala*. The relative abundance of this pollen suggests vast breathtaking flower-filled meadows.

The Younger Dryas period saw a decline of temperatures in Greenland by 4° to 10°C and re-advances of glaciers over much of the temperate Northern Hemisphere. A number of theories have been put forward about the cause. One conjectures that a cluster of comet fragments hit Earth nearly thirteen thousand years ago, causing a catastrophic shift in the climate and the mass extinction of the ice age megafauna. During that time, humans switched from a hunter-gatherer lifestyle to one primarily centered on agriculture and the creation of permanent settlements, maybe in response to the changing environment.

The profound interrelatedness of everything is evident when an alpine herb highlights the evolutionary effects of interplanetary space!

Today, studies are showing that species are becoming extinct at a significantly faster rate than has been the case for millions of years, but even so, extinctions remain relatively rare, giving the impression that the loss of biodiversity is happening only gradually. Nevertheless, the human impact on the diversity of living species is one of the primary attributes of the Anthropocene.

Seed Banks

The reality of biodiversity loss has invoked some creative responses. The phenomenon of survival seed banks is one. A conservative estimate puts the current loss of plant species at a rate that is between a hundred and a thousand times higher than the expected natural extinction rate. Of the approximately eighty thousand flowering plant species, about fifteen thousand species are threatened with extinction from overharvesting and habitat destruction.

Seed banks are increasingly being set up to store the genetic diversity of medicinal plants, preserving the biological and genetic diversity of primarily wild plant species. According to the Food and Agriculture Organization of the United Nations (FAO), in 2010 there were 1,750 gene banks worldwide, representing many millions of plants. One example of such a seed bank is the Svalbard Global Seed Vault, built inside a mountain in permafrost on the Norwegian island of Spitsbergen, 812 miles from the North Pole. The Svalbard vault can store up to 4.5 million varieties of crops and 2.5 billion seeds. It currently houses more than 1.14 million samples of about 6,000 different plant species. The vault provides a safety net in case of loss of diversity in other gene banks, whether due to accident, equipment failures, funding cuts, or natural disasters. Unfortunately, such disasters are surprisingly common. The national seed bank of the Philippines was damaged by flooding and later destroyed by a fire; the seed banks of Afghanistan and Iraq have been lost completely.

Another example is the U.K.'s Millennium Seed Bank, considered to be the most diverse wild plant genetic resource in the world. It features flood-, bomb-, and radiation-proof vaults, with a collection of more than 2.4 billion seeds belonging to about 40,000 species. In addition to preserving Britain's native plant species, it includes collections from 189 countries, so that it stores nearly 16 percent of the world's wild plant species.

In the United States, the National Laboratory for Genetic Resources Preservation in Fort Collins, Colorado, currently stores more than 500,000 samples from 12,000 species, and it has capacity to store 1.5 million samples in total.

The seed banks also contribute to the preservation of indigenous cultures and their plants. The Potato Park, located in Pisac, Peru, an area known as the Sacred Valley of the Incas, is such a place. Managed by local indigenous communities, the park conserves traditional Andean crops including maize and quinoa, but it has a special focus on potatoes. It houses around 2,300 of the 4,000 varieties of potatoes known in the world, and 23 of the 200 wild species of potatoes currently known. Potatoes were first domesticated in this region some 8,000 years ago, near the shores of Lake Titicaca, not far from Pisac.

Climate change will become a much greater threat in the future. Many of the world's poorest people rely on medicinal plants not only as their primary health care option but also as a significant source of income. The potential loss of many medicinal and aromatic plants due to effects of climate change will impact the livelihoods of large numbers of vulnerable people across the world.

Herbalists are acutely aware of the dangers faced by natural populations of healing plants, whether from the uncertainties of climate change, the pressure of land use changes, or overzealous collection by herbalists themselves. The response to these challenges is generally local and regional, as demonstrated by United Plant Savers organization of the United States (see page 180).

Terrestrial Invertebrate Loss

In the twenty-seven years between 1989 and 2016, insect populations declined more than 75 percent in Germany (Hallmann et al. 2017). Worldwide, a 2014 summary of global declines in biodiversity and abundance estimated a 45 percent drop in the abundance of invertebrates, most of which are insects. Loss of insect diversity and abundance will provoke cascading effects on food webs and pollination. Wildlife is dying out due to habitat destruction, overhunting, toxic pollution, invasion by alien species, and climate change. But the ultimate cause of all these factors is humanity.

Earthworms are essential for healthy soil in many parts of the world. However, nonecological agricultural practices have been found to correlate to an 80 percent decline in earthworm populations. This decline is thought to be due to five reasons: soil degradation and destruction of habitat, climate change, biological invasion of nonnative species, poor soil management, and pollutant loading (Maggi and Tang 2021). One can only surmise that these same issues affect populations of all soil organisms.

Freshwater Species Loss

Freshwater habitats are incredibly diverse, with a natural abundance of rivers, lakes, and wetlands. However, some 35 percent of wetlands have been lost in the past fifty years, and only 33 percent of the world's large rivers are still free-flowing. Freshwater species are declining at twice the rate of species located on land or within the ocean. Freshwater vertebrate populations have declined by 83 percent since 1970, and nearly one-third of all freshwater fish are threatened with extinction (WWF 2021, 2022).

Climate Change

Global warming—that is, the rise in the average temperature of the planet—is caused by humans. The size and intensity of climate change is being driven primarily by man-made carbon dioxide emissions. Burning fossil fuels adds greenhouse gases, including carbon dioxide and methane, to the atmosphere. Other inputs come from agriculture, industrial processes, and deforestation. These gases warm the air by absorbing heat and then trapping it near the surface; Earth then takes in more energy from sunlight than it can radiate back into space. Global warming, in turn, has triggered climate change—a plethora of disruptions to the stability of planetary ecology.

The diverse effects of climate change on medicinal plants are starting to become clear. We are seeing not only the expected impacts on plant growth and development but also the corollary impacts on the people who depend upon these herbs for health care. Plants are extremely sensitive to climatic changes. Elevated levels of carbon dioxide, ozone, changing temperature and rainfall, disruption of ecological relationships, and increases in pests and pathogens all influence plant growth. The situation is compounded by human activity, especially overharvesting.

Climate change is altering conditions so that they are no longer ideal—or even survivable—for some species that now inhabit them. Distributions of many medicinal plants are already shifting rapidly toward higher latitudes or elevations. Herbs living in mountain regions are at greatest risk of habitat loss. Alpine meadows, having a rich flora of medicinal plants, are shrinking. Habitat destruction, pollution, and worsening climate change will exacerbate this problem.

A growing recognition concerns herb response to ever-increasing environmental stresses, one of which concerns changes in secondary metabolite metabolism, potentially affecting quality or even safety (Applequist et al. 2020). Decreased potency of a plant medicine might well go unnoticed or might be misinterpreted by a new generation of consumers as inherent lack of efficacy, leading to abandonment of useful plants. Drought stress and high temperatures often increases the concentration of bioactive secondary metabolites, potentially causing increased harm by those that are toxic. Crucially, the resilience that beneficial medicinal plants provide to humans is expected to decline.

Tipping Points

The pageant of human history has brought us to multiple tipping points. A tipping point is the critical threshold in any system beyond which a change—generally unstoppable and self-perpetuating—in the system takes place. Exceeding a tipping point may lead to abrupt and irreversible impacts.

Climate tipping points occur when change in any significant part of the global climate system passes a threshold whereby it becomes a self-perpetuating force that drives a particular climate structure or process into a new pattern, with further impacts developing from there. Global warming, for example, increases the risk of crossing tipping-point thresholds beyond which impacts can't be avoided even if temperatures are later reduced. Some large-scale changes could occur over a short time period, such as a shutdown of certain ocean currents. If those ocean currents diminish significantly, then other climate patterns—temperatures in Europe, for example, or acidification levels in oceans—become disrupted as well.

The numbers are clear, the trends are worrying, and yet we make no meaningful changes. . . .

Societal Collapse

Although herbalism has been present in human life from as long as there have been records, the longevity of the cultures the herbalist found themselves in is another matter. One of the lessons of history is the impermanence of human societies. In a survey of eighty-seven ancient civilizations (from 3000 BCE to 600 CE), the average life span was found to be about 340 years (Kemp 2019). This is surprisingly short.

Virtually all civilizations suffer such a fate, regardless of their size or complexity. The diversity of forms societies evolve into corresponds to the diversity of the ways in which they fail, whether caused by climate change, natural disasters, foreign invasions, mass migration, famine, economic depression, internal strife, or disease outbreaks.

An example would be the Black Death, which killed two hundred million people in the fourteenth century. Consequently, it destabilized most of European society and undermined the system of feudalism and the authority of the Church. Another example would be the introduction of disease to the New World by European colonialism. As much as 90 to 95 percent of the Indigenous American population died from Old World diseases such as smallpox, measles, whooping cough, bubonic plague, malaria, yellow fever, and dengue fever.

A modern reader might dismiss these statistics as being too out-of-date to be useful to a sophisticated, educated, technologically savvy modern population. Yet a 2022 UN report pointed to the increased probability of civilizational collapse as ever more complex interactions between disasters, economic vulnerabilities, and ecosystem failures increase the risk of global collapse. This is the first time the UN has issued a major report finding that existing global policies might be hastening the collapse of human civilization. According to the report, "The human material and ecological footprint is accelerating the rate of change. A potential impact when systemic risks become cascading disasters is that systems are at risk of collapse" (UNDRR 2022, 48).

Existential Risk: Are We Having Fun Yet?

There is an important piece of what might be called "apocalyptic semantics" to clarify. What is an existential risk? A global catastrophic risk is an event that could be damaging on a global scale, even destroying modern civilization. An existential risk is an event that might cause human extinction or drastically curtail humanity's potential (Bostrom 2013).

Some risks that might qualify as globally catastrophic or existential are natural in origin and have caused mass extinctions in the past. Some are man-made, such as a global war, nuclear holocaust, bioterrorism, cyberterrorism, the failure to manage a pandemic, global warming, environmental degradation, extinction of species, human overpopulation, crop failures, and nonsustainable agriculture. Do any of these sound familiar? One could argue that the diversity of the man-made risks is a reflection of the diversity and "success" of technology used as a way of controlling nature.

Ending the "Orgy of Destruction"

Humanity has become a weapon of mass extinction and governments must end the "orgy of destruction," UN Secretary-General António Guterres said at the organization's Biodiversity Conference in 2022. He continued:

> We are out of harmony with nature. In fact, we are playing an entirely different song. Around the world, for hundreds of years, we have conducted a cacophony of chaos, played with instruments of

destruction. Deforestation and desertification are creating waste-lands of once-thriving ecosystems. . . . Our land, water and air are poisoned by chemicals and pesticides, and choked with plastics. . . . The most important lesson we impart to children is to take respon-sibility for their actions. What example are we setting when we our-selves are failing this basic test?

Scientists have been communicating how alarming the situation is for more than fifty years. In 1971, American biologist Barry Commoner argued that the "rate of exploitation of the ecosystem, which generates economic growth, cannot increase indefinitely without overdriving the system and pushing it to the point of collapse" (Commoner 1971, 139). Since then, statements warning of the impending polycrisis have become almost routine. However, the desperation of the situation coupled with despondency about the lack of meaningful response is becoming more evident.

In 1992, the first "World Scientists' Warning to Humanity" high-lighted the dangers of human-caused damage to the biosphere, and to biodiversity overall. The signatories, which including ninety-nine Nobel Prize laureates, called for stabilization of the human population and reduced consumption to avoid environmental catastrophes.

Thirty years later, a second warning underscored the roughly 40 percent increase in global greenhouse gas emissions, despite numer-ous warnings from the Intergovernmental Panel on Climate Change (Ripple et al. 2022). This second warning encouraged scientists to pre-pare discipline-specific papers highlighting the potential detrimental effects of climate change on specific aspects of environmental or human well-being. The diverse scientific community exploring medicinal plants released such a warning in 2020 (Applequist et al. 2020).

Sustainability Goals
Humankind now faces the existential threat of climate change. Increased heat waves, droughts, and apocalyptic wildfires and floods are already affecting billions of people around the globe and causing

potentially irreversible damage to Earth's ecosystems. To avoid the worst effects of climate change, global greenhouse gas emissions will need to peak before 2025 and then decline by 43 percent by 2030, falling to net zero by 2050. Instead, under current voluntary national commitments to climate action, greenhouse gas emissions will rise by nearly 14 percent by 2030. Concurrently, the world is witnessing the largest number of violent conflicts since 1946, with one-quarter of the global population now living in an area affected by conflict. As of May 2022, a record one hundred million people had been forcibly displaced from their homes. The outbreak of war in Ukraine caused food, fuel, and fertilizer prices to skyrocket, disrupted supply chains and global trade, and roiled financial markets, fueling the threat of a global food crisis.

The UN's 2030 Agenda for Sustainable Development, adopted in 2015, presented seventeen goals to be achieved by 2030. These goals are interlinked objectives designed to serve as a shared blueprint for peace and prosperity of people and the planet—in the present and the future. The aim is to lead the world to a healthy, inclusive, and sustainable society, where all people can fulfill their needs while living within our planetary limits. It offers plans and targets for ending poverty and other deprivations hand-in-hand with strategies to improve health and education, reduce inequality, and spur economic growth—all while tackling climate change and working to preserve our oceans and forests. It's a holistic, well-reasoned, evidence-driven, and achievable plan for long-term sustainability. As of a self-imposed accountability progress report in 2022, however, cascading and interlinked crises are putting the 2030 Agenda for Sustainable Development in grave danger, along with humanity's very own survival.

A confluence of crises, dominated by pandemics, climate change, and violent conflicts, are creating spin-off impacts on food and nutrition, health, education, the environment, and peace and security and affecting all of the 2030 Agenda's sustainable development goals. The 2022 accountability report details the reversal of years of progress in eradicating poverty and hunger, improving health and education, providing basic services, and much more.

Among the goals laid out by the 2030 Agenda for Sustainable Development are some for which herbalism can make direct contribution as a crucial tool for resilience. Goal 3, for example, is to ensure healthy lives and promote well-being for all at all ages. Traditional herbalism has an obvious role in that objective. This is a place where herbal (and nutritional) support of health is not only a well-established therapeutic contribution but can be a part of local community empowerment.

However, indirect contributions can be made to most of the other goals. For example, Goal 2 aims to end hunger, achieve food security, and promote sustainable agriculture by doubling agricultural productivity and incomes of small-scale food producers, in particular women, indigenous peoples, family farmers, and pastoralists. Promoting herb cultivation would be an effective contribution with minimal environmental costs.

Goal 5 concerns gender equality and the empowerment of all women. Recognized as a fundamental human right, gender equality is also a precondition for economic growth and prosperity. Economic and social empowerment for women can derive from the skills of herbalism. Which leads to Goal 8, the active promotion of sustained and sustainable economic growth and full and productive employment. This is immediately supported by the decent job creation, entrepreneurship, creativity, and innovation available in the field of herbalism.

UN 2030 Agenda for
Sustainable Development Goals

These goals are an example of the UN at its best. Each goal is not only relevant to the polycrisis but presented in a way that points to very achievable steps toward its attainment. Most significant is the obvious synergy among these goals, a synergy emphasized by the UN as leading to the breadth of positive transformation needed.

Goal 1. End poverty in all its forms everywhere.

Goal 2. End hunger, achieve food security and improved nutrition, and promote sustainable agriculture.

Goal 3. Ensure healthy lives and promote well-being for all at all ages.

Goal 4. Ensure inclusive and equitable quality education and promote lifelong learning opportunities for all.

Goal 5. Achieve gender equality and empower all women and girls.

Goal 6. Ensure availability and sustainable management of water and sanitation for all.

Goal 7. Ensure access to affordable, reliable, sustainable, and modern energy for all.

Goal 8. Promote sustained, inclusive, and sustainable economic growth, full and productive employment, and decent work for all.

Goal 9. Build resilient infrastructure, promote inclusive and sustainable industrialization, and foster innovation.

Goal 10. Reduce inequality within and among countries.

Goal 11. Make cities and human settlements inclusive, safe, resilient, and sustainable.

Goal 12. Ensure sustainable consumption and production patterns.

Goal 13. Take urgent action to combat climate change and its impacts.

Goal 14. Conserve and sustainably use the oceans, seas, and marine resources for sustainable development.

Goal 15. Protect, restore, and promote sustainable use of terrestrial ecosystems, sustainably manage forests, combat desertification, halt and reverse land degradation, and halt biodiversity loss.

Goal 16. Promote peaceful and inclusive societies for sustainable development, provide access to justice for all, and build effective, accountable, and inclusive institutions at all levels.

Goal 17. Strengthen the means of implementation and revitalize the global partnership for sustainable development.

Traditional Ecological Knowledge and Cultural Resilience

The simple skills and knowledge of traditional herbalism are uniquely suited to the challenges ahead. The skills are basic, relevant, accessible, low tech, and minimally impactful, and at the same time personally empowering.

Herbalism and the herbalist in his or her herb garden might at one time have been seen as idyllic hippie agrarianism but can now be recognized as part of a resilient response to a predictable, foreseeable collapse/crisis. In the short term, the skills and knowledge of herbalism can make immense contributions to both emergency response and longer-term recovery, contributing with locally accessible support of community health care. Thus the traditional ecological knowledge (TEK) of basic herbalism being carried by herbalists is more than just the remembrance and continuation of the old ways; it is relevant, accessible, and current—and necessary.

The concept of resilience is insightful here. Resilience refers to the capacity of an individual or system to maintain and renew itself when its viability is threatened. Ecological resilience is the ability of an ecosystem to continue functioning amid and recover from a disturbance. Cultural resilience is the ability of a culture to maintain and develop itself despite adversity or risk. Rather than confronting or battling the challenge, a resilient response focuses on coping.

Human societies have never been more globally interconnected and technologically efficient, while at the same time less resilient—that is, less able to handle, physically and psychologically, the disruptive changes we face in the decades ahead. As natural disasters and wars rip apart societies and as large-scale modernization projects, urbanization, and transnational migration bring about sudden dislocations, the endurance of cultural beliefs, values, practices, and knowledge and their transmission across generations have become significant factors. Cultural continuity is not just an ethnographic concern; it has appreciable, measurable positive benefits for the resilience of human communities. Projects carried out by UNESCO in Haiti, for example, have found that having a vibrant local culture plays an important part in rebuilding a sense of community after disasters.

Authorized, centralized, official herbalism is not the same as TEK. In the cross-fertilization between ecology and sociology, ideas are being clarified that are very helpful here. Who are the carriers by which the knowledge, experience, and practice of managing a local ecosystem and its services are captured, stored, revived, and transmitted through time?

The landscapes that facilitate such social memory have been called biocultural refugia. Refugia were originally defined as geographical areas of relative ecological stability that enabled long-term survival during periods of glaciation. However, *biocultural* refugia also carry knowledge about the practical management of food production while maintaining biodiversity and ecosystem viability.

TEK, such as herbalism, is the key to sustainable stewardship of any cultural landscape. It contains the cumulative and evolving body of knowledge, practices, and beliefs held by communities about their relations with the ecosystems in which they are embedded (Barthel, Crumley, and Svedin 2013).

Herbalism, with its intimate relationship with the land and the people on it, has been a vibrant and still extant worldwide biocultural refugia. The diversity of ecological, geographical, and cultural conditions for the collection, cultivation, and preparation of medicinal plants is reflected in the rich tapestry of ethnobotany—of people's herbalism. But the concept of herbalism as a biocultural refugia is much more than the regional history of herbalism or the picture of plant use around the world being explored by ethnobotanists today.

Biocultural refugia can be viewed as pockets of social-ecological memory. These refugia—widely varied, place specific, ever evolving—produce and protect interlinked biological and cultural diversity. But biocultural refugia can be dominated or even swiftly wiped out, as is occurring now on a grand scale, and the TEK that supports these refugia is at risk worldwide. TEK is highly adaptive and flexible, but no knowledge system is sustainable without people to carry on its practices. Ubiquitous industrialization is rapidly eroding the use and memory of such practices, treating them as "obsolete." Powerful government and "professional" organizations have imposed standards, tools, and metrics that do not have a place for the "old ways." Globalization suppresses the languages, religions, habits, and livelihoods of communities everywhere, eroding their traditions and TEK. Traditional practices, along with their stewardship of interlinked social-ecological systems, are being discarded in an ongoing generational amnesia.

Despite the generalized worldwide trend of TEK erosion, substantial pockets of TEK persist in both developing and developed countries. Herbalism, in its often-bewildering array of manifestation, is one of them. Herbalism has not been discarded by the people—simply by the dominant culture.

TEK of how to find, grow, harvest, and use particular plants probably predates the evolution of agro-biodiversity in any particular geographical areas. This TEK of our deep past and the evolving traditional medical/herbal strategies that were successful were passed on through our cultural collective memory, maintained through social interaction in families, communities, settlements, professional groups, and even religious practice.

Memory carriers of TEK evolve. They can be immaterial, like meanings and ideas, and physical, like artifacts, landraces, and landscape features. They can be rituals, oral traditions, written accounts, and self-organized systems of rules. They continue to transmit TEK long after the people who created them are gone. Memory carriers are emergent structures; they are continually revived through the incorporation of novel experiences. Herbalists have cultivated memory carriers of TEK in a number of ways: names of plants and remedies; songs and stories, passed from one generation to the next; visual and other mnemonic cues left in landscapes, monuments, and objects; the embodiment of everyday practice taught through dance or the cadence of work; every written record, a "message in a bottle" from the past.

The whole gamut of skills and knowledge that are encompassed by the phrase *traditional ecological knowledge* can strengthen the capacity of societies to deal with disturbances under conditions of uncertainty and change. The herbal health care component of this wonderfully empowering gift of the ancestors is potentially complex, but at the same time very simple. The techniques and insights are readily accessible to the nonprofessional while also being respectable to a range of professional elites, whether medical or scientific.

9

What Is a
Simple Herbalist to Do?

In the face of all this apocalyptic feculence, what is a simple herbalist to do? What role can herbalism play in these trying times, let alone those to come? Can herbalism help culture find its way to a viable future while the "system" thrashes about?

Given the currently unfolding panoply of crises, it seems safe to say that at least the next hundred years will be characterized by multiple interlinked crises, the nature of which can be debated (and will probably be surprising), but their impact will be catastrophic. Herbalism cannot meaningfully address these crises or their causes, but it could have a unique and possibly essential influence on cultural viability in the near future. The immediate concern needs to focus on emergency response and crisis management. Whether officially recognized or not, herbalism is a key component of the whole panoply of national health care, and it can greatly augment community resilience.

The chronic inadequacy of the modern health care system, alongside humanity's untenable relationship with the world, was highlighted by the panicked, divisive global response to the COVID-19 pandemic. Even more profound health care challenges and chaos are en route, fueled by the multifactorial nature of the polycrisis. But herbalism can ameliorate the trauma. Out of the maelstrom rises the possibility of the renewal and rebirth of a planetary community that has learned to live in harmony with life, with green sensibilities informing all that humans do.

Support Grassroots Medicine

When prescription drugs become too expensive for most of the world—because petroleum reserves have been exhausted, climate disruptions have thrown production and distribution networks into chaos, the resources from which the drugs are made are depleted, and other factors yet to be known—the knowledge and skills of the herbalist will no longer be fringe. Even today, as the collapse proceeds, herbalism is reemerging, awakening to its role in building community resilience and resistance to humanity's ravaging of the planet.

One of the key signs of herbalism's vibrant reemergence as a medicine of the people is the rapid manifestation of a true grassroots health care system. Health care activists have started to build a postindustrial self-help medical system that will more than fill the gaps of the collapsing health care system, and community herbalism is an integral part of this movement. Of course, herbalism does not replace the need for modern medicine, with its surgical miracles and occasionally life-saving drugs, but it is absolutely the basis of good home health care and wellness medicine.

As the health care paradigm shifts toward more holistic perspectives, insights arising from the traditional ecological knowledge (TEK) of herbalism are being validated and increasingly valued. In other words, the foundation for socially relevant postindustrial health care is being laid by herbalists of the modern herbal renaissance! See "It Takes a Village" (page 203) for some real-world examples of ways in which herbalists are supporting grassroots medicine.

Seek and Foster Educational Pathways

The past century of technological and scientific triumphalism in the West has almost eradicated our cultural memory of herbal TEK, leaving most people reliant on an increasingly "professionalized," bureaucratic, regulation-reliant system when it comes to managing their own health care. With the coming polycrisis, as even just the single crisis of COVID-19 showed us, this system will be overwhelmed. Acknowledging this highlights the need for education and practical training in herbalism, for both communities at large and aspiring healers. Unfortunately, Western culture is suffering from an herbal drought, especially in terms of the pathways that may lead to becoming an herbalist. Our bereft education systems are of no help in laying the foundations of herbal literacy. Recognizing this lack, the herbal community has created its own paths.

Northeast School of Botanical Medicine

Northeast School of Botanical Medicine, based in Ithaca, New York, aims to ready students for the challenging work of being community-focused herbalists. Founded and run by 7Song, one of the few herbalists acknowledging the polycrisis in his teachings, the Resources portion of his website offers an abundance of empowering articles and handouts, including checklists for different emergency situations and guidelines for dynamic involvement in street and protest medicine. 7Song is also the director of holistic medicine for the Ithaca Free Clinic and assists others who are interested in bringing herbal medicine into free clinics nationwide.

The instructional environment for herbally relevant learning has transformed in recent years through the work of countless herbalists sharing their skills and knowledge and honing their teaching skills. People's medicine has given birth to people's education, as herbalists have taken on the task of introducing herbalism to their communities and training the next generation of practitioners. The wonderful diversity of people involved, the cultures they represent, the plants they dance with, and their personal experience are reflected in the manifold ways in which herbal education has developed. This array of educational pathways into herbalism is the epitome of a grassroots movement meeting the monolith of mainstream culture. Depending on your perspective, it can be seen as either a wonderful manifestation of people power or a multicar pileup!

The dearth of accredited schools offering herbal education does not imply incompetence or inadequacy in the field but is simply a reflection of the dominant culture ignoring herbalism. From an herbalist's perspective, this might be a good thing. The lack of central authority has led to the need for herbal teachers to create and teach their own curricula, material reflecting their personal interests and experience, and what was at one time an educational desert has bloomed into a fascinating ecology of schools and teachers. They cover different aspects of the use of medicinal plants, with different levels of education and in a variety of forms. This has led to a wonderfully diverse array of educational options, from basic community herbalism to increasingly technical phytotherapy.

Herbalism is simple and easily available, but being an herbalist involves skills, knowledge, and experience. Anyone interested in beginning or furthering their herbal education should look to experienced herbalists and the schools they have created. The American Herbalists Guild maintains an up-to-date guide to the most recent offerings from its members. See "Educational Resources" (page 215) for a list of recommended courses and programs.

Prepare for Emergencies

The past few years have been a rapid education in emergency response for many people, with an apparently never-ending spectacle of fires, floods, pandemics, hurricanes, police riots, white supremacists, Nazis going mainstream, anti-vaxxers . . . The use of herbal remedies in such stressful times has much to commend it. They not only offer well-validated health benefits but also engender the empowering experience of personal agency.

Though basic herbal skills have been part of the human experience for many thousands of years, they have been largely forgotten in the modern world. Knowing the herbs and their healing properties is but a small amount of the body of knowledge available to us. Of course herbalists must be knowledgeable and skillful to be of use to our local communities, but true resilience also necessitates the reclamation of our larger community: the family of herbalists and our place in the world. Herbalists responding to crises and emergency situations do not need permission. The basis here is people power—real grassroots activism! The core need in preparing for emergencies is for us to stand up and be seen as herbalists and as lovers of herbs.

Beginning Steps

Pragmatic steps in preparing for emergencies might include the following.

Learning

This first step will come easily to today's herbalist! Spend time learning about the herbs and the traditional skills of herbalism. Becoming grounded in such skills and knowledge will prepare and equip you for emergencies. Similarly, becoming familiar with the human body in health and illness will illuminate the relevant basics of health care.

Cultivating

Not all herbalists are spontaneous gardeners! If (like me) the garden is not your natural environment, take the plunge and grow a few herbs that do not pose a gardening challenge and have relevant first aid applications. If you have no space for a garden, even something as simple and useful as a window box growing chamomile is a good place to start.

We learn by doing, so plan to use what you grow to make some form of herbal remedy.

Making

Make your own simple herbal formulations, whether medicinal, cosmetic, culinary, or fun! Take your time, and learn from your mistakes (there will be many!). Ideally you will find a teacher who can introduce you to and steer you through your medicine-making journey. If that is not a possibility, there are some excellent books written by experienced herbalists that guide beginners through the process. Examples are listed on the following page. A good goal here would be to create and stock a home herbal first aid kit.

Good Guides to Making Herbal Medicines

The Herbal Medicine-Maker's Handbook: A Home Manual, by James Green

Making Plant Medicine, by Richo Cech

The Modern Herbal Dispensatory: A Medicine-Making Guide, by Thomas Easley and Steven Horne

Rosemary Gladstar's Herbal Recipes for Vibrant Health: 175 Teas, Tonics, Oils, Salves, Tinctures, and Other Natural Remedies for the Entire Family, by Rosemary Gladstar

Herbal First Aid

First aid, traditionally defined, is simply emergency care or treatment given in the event of an accident or illness. It's doing what's needed to handle minor injuries or to stabilize a person in severe distress until they can be handed off to a higher level of care. "Herbal" first aid is simply first aid that relies on herbs for their medicinal effects. An excellent primer on this vital topic is *Herbal Medic: A Green Beret's Guide to Emergency Medical Preparedness and Natural First Aid*, by Sam Coffman. It covers basic first aid for issues such as wounds, burns, bruises, and sprains but also fevers, mild infections, coughs, sore throats, nasal congestion, pain, anxiety, and digestive problems.

A first aid kit is a collection of supplies and equipment used to give immediate medical treatment, principally treating injuries and other mild or moderate problems. There is a wide variation in the content of first aid kits based on the knowledge and experience of those putting them together. An herbal first aid kit is simply a first aid kit using herbal components among its tools.

The lack of commercially available herbal first aid kits might be seen as problematic but is often the impetus for learning and applying basic herbal skills. The creation of a personal first aid kit is often one of the first tasks assigned to a student of herbalism.

When you're considering the items you'll stock in your first aid kit, knowing the pros and cons of the various forms of herbal medicines becomes essential. Should the herbs in your kit be fresh, dried, or powdered in capsules? Should the extracts be tinctures or glycerites, and what base is best for ointments? The answer to all of these questions is: It depends!

For example, tinctures are concentrated medicines with a very long shelf life. They should be stored in dark glass bottles to protect them from light exposure, which can degrade components. The dose is usually small, from a few drops up to five milliliters, and can be taken straight or mixed with water or juice. That means a first aid kit doesn't need any great volume of tinctures, and it's easy to administer them in a range of situations.

Another notable detail is that tinctures extract all water- and alcohol-soluble constituents from an herb, while water extracts such as teas will have none of the alcohol-soluble constituents and glycerites will be somewhere in between. The overridingly important point is that glycerites have a much shorter shelf life than tinctures, meaning they might ferment or "go off" easily. That said, the constituent glycerol, the basis of glycerites, poses none of hazards that the alcohol in tinctures does. Glycerites similarly pose none of the taste burden of tinctures—they are neither pungent nor bitter and are generally well received by patients. Glycerites also are safe even for very young children and during pregnancy (provided, of course, that the herbs used to make them are also safe).

Thus the answer of "it depends" is frustratingly accurate. But let the frustration prompt a search for the answer. The writings of herbalists is the first place to look. The titles listed on the facing page are excellent handbooks that I recommend without reservation, written as they are by expert medicine makers.

Stocking a First Aid Kit

Basic Supplies

Medical adhesive tape (at least 1 inch wide)

Medical/surgical tape

Elastic wrap bandages

Sterile gauze in different sizes

Hemostatic (blood-stopping) gauze

Assorted adhesive bandages (fabric preferred)

Blister treatments (such as moleskin)

Superglue

Rubber tourniquet

Finger splint

Flexible padded aluminum splint (aka SAM splint)

Instant cold packs

Eye shield or pad

Eyewash solution

Cotton balls and cotton-tipped swabs

Plastic bags, assorted sizes

Safety pins, assorted sizes

Thermometer

Fine-point metal tweezers

Bandage scissors

#11 scalpel with extra blades

20 cc irrigation syringe

USP-grade charcoal

Nitrile gloves

Alcohol wipes

Hand sanitizer

Cleansing pads with topical anesthetic

CPR mask

Bee-sting kit

Tick remover

Rehydration salts

Glucose or other sugar (to treat hypoglycemia)

Medical waste bag (plus box for sharp items)

Emergency heat-reflecting blanket

Waterproof matches

Small waterproof flashlight or headlamp and extra batteries

Notepad and waterproof writing instrument

Solar charger for cell phones

First aid manual

Phone numbers for local emergency services, emergency road service providers, and poison help line

. . . .

Primary Herbs

These herbs are broadly useful and readily available, making them excellent components of a first aid kit. For information on their uses and
dosage guidelines, see "Some Core Herbs to Know" on page 186. In
terms of which forms of these herbs to stock in your kit—fresh, dried,
capsules, ointments, tinctures, glycerites, and so on—the answer is, as
noted above, it depends. Range of use, ease of use, portability, and shelf
life are certainly important factors to consider.

Arnica	Shepherd's purse
Boneset	Skullcap
Calendula	St. John's wort
Chamomile	Thyme
Chickweed	Valerian
Comfrey	Witch hazel
Echinacea	Yarrow
Meadowsweet	

. . . .

Additional Herbs to Consider

A complete list of herbs that are very useful in first aid situations
would be very long—and a source of endless debate among herbalists!
However, here is a brief list of additional herbs to explore.

Black walnut hull and leaf	Oregon grape root
Burdock root	Passionflower
Cornsilk	Prickly ash bark/berry
Elder flower	Prickly pear
Ginger	Spilanthes leaf
Horsetail	Uva ursi
Lobelia	Wild oats
Marshmallow root and leaf	Wood betony
Nettles	Yerba mansa

Herbal first aid products and complete kits can be purchased from the online shops of Herbal First Aid Gear and Mountain Rose Herbs. When stocking your kit or cabinet, always confirm that the herbal components are appropriate for your needs, and if not, make your own.

Build a Resilient Medicine Chest

Looking beyond the basic first aid kit, a more comprehensive herbal medicine chest for community health care might be considered essential for resilient well-being in times of crisis and challenge. The term "medicine chest" generally means some sort of container used for storing medicines or first aid supplies. Here, it connotes simply a collection of herbs and formulas that address a range of common health issues and are held at the ready, able to be put into use whenever the need arises. A trained herbalist would have a much more extensive medicine chest than most people, but any person with basic herbal literacy can make good use of common medicinal herbs to soothe, heal, and comfort all manner of everyday health complaints. Given the concerns for our future, this empowerment and resilience should not be underestimated.

A challenge herbalists sometimes face is determining which system of herbalism to use as a basis for selecting herbs and identifying conditions to treat. We are blessed by a cornucopia, from the profoundly holistic systems of ayurveda and traditional Chinese medicine to the reductionist approach of allopathic medicine. Acknowledging this diversity, herbalists should avoid what might be described as herbal mixing and matching (some might call it cultural appropriation), which risks losing sight of the unique therapeutic perspectives offered by the herbal traditions of the world. The material below uses the framework of eclectic Western herbalism the author was trained in.

Like all medicines, herbal medicines must be used in the context of addressing factors such as diet, lifestyle, and emotional, mental, and spiritual health, all of which must be considered within a socio-economic context. The issues raised by these considerations, as well the theoretic underpinnings of herb selection, are not explored here. While a coherent, rational theoretical model underlies the condensed suggestions below, here is not the place to present the conceptual details. I explore them further in my books *The Herbal Handbook: A User's Guide to Medical Herbalism* and *Medical Herbalism: The Science and Practice of Herbal Medicine*. Another good resource is naturopathic physician Jill Stansbury's five-volume textbook series Herbal Formularies for Health Professionals, which is in my opinion the best modern examination of formulation to achieve focused therapeutic outcomes. She covers the plethora of issues that need to be addressed in formulating for digestion and elimination, circulation and respiration, endocrinology, neurology and pain management, and finally immunology, orthopedics, and otolaryngology.

The Plants

Get to know the herbs you will use in your medicine chest. Read all you can about them, grow them, eat them, talk to them. Knowing the herbs means knowing where they live, so get to know them in their favorite habitats. Get to know your local habitats and identify what common herbs grow where. Even if you are not intending to wildcraft, be familiar with and follow the ethical guidelines for collection (see page 181) or, more importantly, how to be with the herbs ethically. It is often our very humanity that gets in the way of communing with nature.

Wild Collection vs. Cultivation

Herbs can be either cultivated or collected from the wild. However, *can* is not the same as *should*. The matrix of considerations ranges from ecological, economic, and political to spiritual and ethical. Recognizing the natural world's gift of medicinal plants should not give free rein to the malign tendency of capitalism to assume that anything free is free to be used or taken.

There are too many people needing health care to sustain the collection of wild populations of medicinal plants. This means that herbs must be primarily cultivated, and that should be organic cultivation. Although there are no studies to support these statements, we must look to the precautionary principle, whose central component calls for taking proactive steps in the face of uncertainty—for anticipating harm and working to prevent it before it occurs. It might be interpreted as the evolution of the ancient medical principle of "first, do no harm," in this case applied to institutions and institutional decision-making processes rather than individuals.

The precautionary principle tells us that medicinal plants should be cultivated, thus ensuring supply while mitigating collection pressure on wild populations. Wildcrafting should be saved for a last resort.

This stance is not specifically related to the identity of the herb. In fact, concerns about the ecological status of any particular herb are the least of my worries. I am greatly encouraged by the quality and depth of attention being given to the conservation of wild medicinal plants. The assessment of the whole panoply of factors affecting their collection, from their endangered status to sustainability to adulteration concerns, is well in hand. From my point of view, the most important (but often most difficult) issue is whether traditional knowledge of and experience with plants are being respected.

A subtly different point is the assessment of whether the collection is causing ecological damage to plant communities. Does wildcrafting contribute to soil compaction and erosion? Are we paying attention to the impact of wildcrafting on insects in light of dramatic decline in insect populations worldwide? What is the impact of local transport to and from the collection sites? How is human encroachment on wild sites detracting from the natural ecology at those sites? These and other forms of damage caused simply by human activity need to be taken into account.

Whether any of this is seen as problematic depends largely on personal worldview. There are no certainties, and each situation must be assessed on its merits, but to be clear: I choose to question the morality, ethics, and sanity of such things. The lust for product and addiction to the profit it offers is nothing to support. I see it as a very personal ecological crime each of us commits as we do our part in facilitating such trade. We must each choose where we stand on this, or the culture will choose for us.

This is a place where ecological considerations and the constraints they may lead to will have an immediate impact on herbalists. It is also where things get political, with all the messy emotions that implies! It rapidly comes down to whether we take climate issues seriously or use them as convenient ways to avoid and deflect, contorting ourselves to stay in our comfort zone. Humanity, which of course includes herbalists, is facing the repercussions of viewing the world as a resource.

In identifying the contributions herbalism can make to humanity's transition out of the role of despoiler and into a role as a family member, it would be ironic to perpetuate the abuse by default. Empowering people with the tools of herbal health care in order to support resilience in times of crisis must not harm the environment in which the herbs grow.

In light of regional availability as well as locally cultivated herbs, there is rarely a need for expensive or exotic herbs. The occasionally exorbitant price of medicinal herbs reflects scarcity or the costs of commerce; it is not an indication of quality. Because of the absurdities of globalized markets and supply chains, much commercial chamomile comes from Egypt. Egyptian chamomile is cultivated and processed to the highest quality, but what about its carbon footprint? The environmental costs of international supply chains may be rapidly approaching levels that challenge the primacy of quality in purchasing decisions. A difficult and painful issue arises here: Does human health outweigh environmental health in these times of polycrisis?

As much of the pressure faced by populations of wild herbs comes from the herbalists themselves, an herbal way of dealing with the problem is appropriate. If an herb of concern is being collected for its specific therapeutic properties, then an herbalist can and should identify other herbs—prioritizing those that can be cultivated rather than wildcrafted—that have those same properties. Of course the properties of two different species will never be identical, but by careful selection it is usually possible to replace an at-risk plant with another plant (or a combination of plants) that have the same effect. (See "Making Sense of Herbal Diversity," on page 49, for some examples of plants with similar actions.)

A look at the ideas of Northern Californian herbalist Jane Bothwell illustrates how an herbalist would reduce the risk to at-risk plants. Bothwell offers the example of black cohosh (*Actaea racemosa*), a well-known North

American medicinal plant (and one of the most important contributions North America has made to phytotherapy worldwide). Black cohosh might be prescribed for its anti-inflammatory properties, but it is considered at risk in the wild. If an herbalist wants to avoid using the herb for conservation reasons, there are many other anti-inflammatories to choose from. Black cohosh also gently relaxes muscles, which together with the anti-inflammatory action might explain the herb's benefits in rheumatism. If the anti-inflammatory used as a replacement is chamomile, there is a complication. Although an excellent anti-inflammatory, chamomile does not relax strained muscles the way black cohosh does. To achieve the desired effects, chamomile might be combined with cramp bark, a non-sedating muscle relaxant. In this way the herbalist has conserved black cohosh but maintained efficacy in the prescription.

United Plant Savers

The herbal community has responded to threats of overcollection of medicinal plants in an inspiring grassroots way. United Plant Savers (UpS) was formed in 1995 with a mission to "protect native medicinal plants of the United States and Canada and their native habitats while ensuring an abundant supply of medicinal plants for generations for come." In the face of habitat loss and overharvesting, UpS is coordinating efforts to preserve native medicinal plant populations.

UpS maintains a list of herbs regarded as the most vulnerable to overharvesting (the at-risk list) and those less vulnerable but still of great concern (the watch list). A spectrum of factors making the herbs sensitive to human activity were considered, including market analysis, habitat specificity, impacts of harvest, and lack of techniques or material for large-scale cultivation. The initial UpS at-risk list included fourteen herbs, and the watch list included seventeen. As of this writing, the at-risk list has grown to twenty-three herbs:

American ginseng	Bloodroot
Arnica	Blue cohosh
Black cohosh	Cascara sagrada

Echinacea	Osha
Eyebright	Peyote
False unicorn root	Slippery elm
Gentian	Sundew
Goldenseal	True unicorn root
Goldthread	Wild indigo
Kava kava	Wild yam
Lady's slipper orchid	Yerba mansa
Lobelia	

Find the most up-to-date versions of the at-risk and to-watch lists on the United Plant Savers website.

These lists fill a unique role in plant conservation. Many agencies have created at-risk lists for plants and wildlife; for example, the U.S. Endangered Species Act protects the very rarest of species, and NatureServe provides a standard ranking system used by all U.S. states to score plant species based on rarity and abundance. None, however, consider issues specific to medicinal plants, as UpS does. The organization is not promoting a moratorium on the use of these herbs but, instead, initiating programs designed to preserve them.

Ethical Wildcrafting

Ethical wildcrafting is the practice of harvesting wild plants conscientiously, avoiding any damage to the population or their habitat. An ethical wildcrafter will not harvest in a way that kills the plant when taking just a part of it will do, will not collect more than is needed, and will not take more than the habitat can support so that the harvest remains sustainable.

For at-risk species, ethical wildcrafting usually means not harvesting from wild specimens. For example, ginseng has been so overharvested in parts of the United States to the point that the plant's very survival is threatened and several states have had to implement ginseng management programs. Ethical wildcrafters will not harvest ginseng. United Plant Savers maintains an updated list of at-risk plant species in the United States and Canada; even beginning wildcrafters should know it well. A simple rule of thumb: When in doubt, don't pick it.

When wildcrafting, the same intention and conscientiousness brought to the plants should be applied to the habitat in which they grow. The health of the land is, of course, crucial to not only the health of any herb collected but also the health of the people who use that herb. Human activity exposes the natural world to an astonishing plethora of toxic pollutants. An ethical wildcrafter should avoid collection sites near busy roads, abandoned industrial or military sites, and so on. If collecting near running water, make sure it is not polluted. Be gentle and delicate when passing through the land! Are there rare, threatened, endangered, or sensitive plants growing nearby, not just when you are there but at any time of the year?

Know how to identify the medicinal plants you want, but also how to tell them apart from similar-looking plants. Never collect more than 10 percent of any wild plant stand. Allow the oldest and largest plants to remain; their genes are the hardiest and most successful, so it's important for the health of their species that they continue to reproduce.

Other concerns include botanical, ecological, and even legal specifics. For example, is permission needed to collect herbs at a specific site? Never trespass for herbs. Assess the effect of harvesting on all the plants in the collection site and on the land in general. Is any cleanup needed?

Practitioners of ethical wildcrafting emphasize the importance of attitude and state of mind, believing that it's essential to strengthening the symbiotic relationship that exists between the herbalist and the earth. Wildcrafting is less about the plants harvested than it is a commitment to deepening a connection to the natural landscape and taking responsibility for its regeneration.

Botanical Sanctuaries

United Plant Savers (UpS) has been instrumental in the establishment of botanical sanctuaries around the country. These sanctuaries are much more than the traditional botanic gardens, as important as those are. Botanical sanctuaries are places that affirm the healing matrix these plants are a part of—the matrix of relationships characteristic of the ecology of plants and animals embraced by their unique environment. Such sanctuaries provide refuge, a much-needed haven for the plants to thrive, recognizing that as plants thrive, all life thrives, including humans. To quote Rosemary Gladstar, cofounder of UpS:

> When we think of botanical sanctuaries, one often envisions large tracts of land, generally owned by a non-profit, private land trust, or government agency, not something that we as individuals can create. But a botanical sanctuary has little to do with size or own-ership, and much more to do with relationship and intention. It is about good stewardship practices, a relationship that takes into account the natural resources of the land and its native habi-tats and inhabitants; it is about restoring the sacred relationship between people and land. (Gladstar, n.d.).

The UpS Sanctuary Network supports its members in creating these sanctuaries on their own land, with more than 214 botanical sanctuaries in North America to date. At the heart of this network is the Goldenseal Sanctuary, a 370-acre farm located in the Appalachian foothills of southeastern Ohio. Uniquely rich environmental conditions make it a natural refuge for wild medicinal plants, including more than 500 species of plants, 120 species of trees, and 200 species of fungi. Half of the at-risk species recognized by UpS thrive on this land. It is wonder-ful example of the herbal community not only recognizing the problem caused by overharvesting and habitat destruction, but taking on the job of doing something about it.

Bioregional Herbalism

Though my suggestion is to avoid wildcrafting during this time of human-caused environmental pressure on plants, there will always be exceptions. The ideal of letting the land and plants recuperate must be tempered with the needs of alleviating illness and the reality of the herb garden. There may not be enough of a particular herb ready for harvesting or of a quality that is appropriate for health care, but the abundance of the natural world can usually fulfill the herbalist's needs. To access this healing abundance requires knowing what grows naturally in your area and how to gather herbs in an ecologically sound way (see page 181).

How do we access the knowledge and experience of those who know the medicinal uses of local wild plants? While the internet, journals, and regional ethnobotany and herb books are good places to begin, we can dig deeper. Here in North America, we should consider historical writings about Indigenous American uses and ethnobotany. A wealth of material on medicinal plants used by Indigenous Americans was collected in the eighteenth and nineteenth centuries and published in the annual reports of the Smithsonian Institution. Local historical societies often have information in their libraries about local ethnobotany. Ideally, ask members of local (or once local, in the case of peoples dispossessed of their land) Indigenous tribes about their herbal knowledge, experience, and history.

It can come as a surprise that there are local sources of herbal information other than herb stores! It's worth getting creative when trying to identify bioregionally unique medicinal plants. Published information may be in books on local geography or local history, memoirs, or even Victorian pharmacy collections. Historical writings by local herbalists were often self-published and may be found only in regional libraries. School and university libraries often have collections of local or regional material that contains herbal insights. These cornucopias of herbal wisdom are well worth searching for.

The same holds true for herbarium collections. An herbarium is a collection of preserved plant specimens that are stored and catalogued along with associated data used for scientific study. A competent herbarium specimen will have, in addition to botanical, ecological, and taxonomic information, details on the way the plant was used. Herbarium collections are held and maintained in a number of different locations—from botany departments at schools and universities to local and regional governments.

Identifying Regional Stocks of Medicinal Plants

As we work to build a resilient community medicine chest, our goal is to minimize social suffering in the face of crisis. This leads us to socialized herbalism! I mean this in a very positive sense. The basis of herbalism is mutual aid. In times of urgent need, there might be justification for requisitioning medicinal plants from whatever stocks are available locally. (Of course, this concept raises challenging social issues, which won't be explored here.)

A crucial step is to identify existing stocks of herbs actually present regionally. In addition to sustainable wild collection, there are a number of sources to investigate. The obvious ones are herb gardens, whether private, commercial, civic, university, school, or hospital. What plants do they grow, and what medicinal properties do those plants possess? In what quantities are they grown?

Regionally, there may be manufacturers or wholesalers of herbal products that will have meaningful stocks available. Retail stores such as herb stores and supermarkets may also carry some herbs and herbal products.

Practitioners of the various manifestations of herbalism will also have some stocks—and of course vital knowledge and skills. This might include herbalists, clinical phytotherapists, naturopaths, homeopaths, traditional Chinese medicine practitioners, doctors, osteopaths, chiropractors, and especially pharmacists.

The goal is a contribution to the greater good, not the promotion of an herbal agenda, while at the same time taking care not to support the intellectual imperialism of the dominant culture or the health fascism of miracle cures. So whom do we inform about the potential herbal contribution to emergency response? What government bodies (and real people!) might be told of local herbal resources? Examples might include county emergency response personnel, FEMA, paramedics, pharmacists, practitioner groups (all modalities), and school nurses. They also should include local mutual-aid activist groups such as advocates for the homeless, chapters of Food Not Bombs, and service-oriented neighborhood or church groups.

An important cofactor of this effort would be spreading the word about the skills and resources herbalists contribute. Utilizing the opportunities opened through social media, the internet in general, and especially desktop publishing is fundamental to improving community resilience through education and resource sharing. Guides to the regionally available herbs, their preparation, and their use, by and for local communities, are in themselves empowering.

Apothecary Kits

A major contribution to community resilience would be the distribution of apothecary garden kits, sets of medicinal plant seeds that will grow with minimal gardening skills. The seed sets should be accompanied by guides to cultivation, harvesting, and the preparation and use of the herbs. Many commercial medicinal garden kits are available online with different selections of plants. To select an appropriate kit, focus on finding one with the plants most relevant to your specific needs.

Some Core Herbs to Know

The plants listed here have been selected for their availability, ease of use, and minimal safety concerns. These herbs are widely used by the herbal community in North America, so you will find them discussed in most modern herb books.

Arnica (*Arnica montana*)

Part used: Flower heads

Actions: Anti-inflammatory, vulnerary

Indications: Although this herb should not be taken internally, as it is potentially toxic, it is one of the best external remedies for healing bruises and sprains and relieving muscular rheumatic pain. It may be used externally wherever there is pain or inflammation on the skin. The homeopathic preparation of arnica is entirely safe to take internally, making it easy to take advantage of its homeopathic indications, which include bruises, sprains, muscle aches, wound healing, superficial phlebitis, joint pain, and inflammation from insect bites.

Dose: Apply arnica externally (on unbroken skin) as needed.

Boneset (*Eupatorium perfoliatum*)

Part used: Aerial parts

Actions: Antispasmodic, bitter, diaphoretic, laxative

Indications: Boneset is one of the best remedies for influenza symptoms. It will speedily relieve aches and pains as well as aid the body in dealing with fever.

Dose: Boneset is best prepared as a hot tea (infusion); steep 1 to 2 teaspoons of the dried herb per cup of water and drink three times a day. In cases of fever or flu, drink the tea every half hour.

Calendula (*Calendula officinalis*)

Parts used: Flower petals and flower heads

Actions: Anti-inflammatory, antimicrobial, astringent, emmenagogue, lymphatic, vulnerary

Indications: Calendula is one of the best herbs for treating localized skin irritations. It may be used safely for all cases of skin inflammation, whether due to infection or physical damage such as wounds, bruises, or strains. It will also be of benefit for slow-healing wounds and is ideal for first aid treatment of minor burns.

Dose: Apply externally as needed in the form of an ointment (see page 198), poultice, or compress.

Chamomile (*Matricaria chamomilla*)

Part used: Flowering tops

Actions: Anti-inflammatory, antimicrobial, antispasmodic, bitter, carminative, nervine, vulnerary

Indications: Chamomile is probably the most widely used relaxing nervine herb in the Western world. It relaxes and tones the nervous system and is especially valuable in cases where anxiety and tension produce digestive symptoms such as gas, colic pains, or even ulcers. It is useful for easing all types of stress and anxiety-related problems. It is also very gentle and safe; used as an addition to the bath, it will help anxious children or teething infants.

Dose: Chamomile can be used fresh or dried. For an infusion, steep

2 teaspoons of the dried herb per cup of water and drink three times a day. The tincture is an excellent way of ensuring that the plant components are extracted and available for the body; take 1 to 4 milliliters three times a day.

Chickweed (*Stellaria media*)

Part used: Aerial parts

Actions: Anti-inflammatory, antipruritic, vulnerary

Indications: Chickweed is commonly used as an external remedy for itching and irritation. It is especially helpful for relieving these symptoms when caused by eczema or psoriasis.

Dose: To ease itching, add a handful or two of the fresh herb to your bathwater (in a cloth sachet, if preferred).

Comfrey (*Symphytum officinale*)

Parts used: Roots and leaves

Actions: Anti-inflammatory, demulcent, vulnerary

Indications: Comfrey's impressive wound-healing properties come partly from its constituent allantoin, a compound that stimulates cell proliferation and so augments wound healing. The herb may be used externally to speed wound healing with minimal scar tissue formation. In fact, comfrey works so well and quickly that caution should be observed when using it with very deep wounds, as the external application of comfrey can lead to tissue forming over the wound before it has healed deeper down, possibly leading to abscesses.

Dose: Apply externally liberally and often in the form of a poultice, compress, lotion, or any other form of medical skin application. The active constituent that promotes skin healing is water soluble so oil or salve forms of comfrey might be less effective.

Echinacea (*Echinacea* spp.)

Part used: Roots

Actions: Antimicrobial

Indications: Echinacea is one of the best herbal remedies available to help the body rid itself of microbial infections. It is often effective against both bacterial and viral attacks. In conjunction with other herbs, it can be used to treat any infection in the body. For example, in combination with yarrow it will effectively stop cystitis. It is especially useful for infections of the upper respiratory tract such as laryngitis and tonsillitis and for catarrhal conditions of the nose and sinuses. It can be used externally in the form of a salve to help septic sores and wounds.

Dose: For a decoction, use 1 to 2 teaspoons of the root per cup of water and drink three times a day. For the tincture, take 1 to 4 milliliters three times a day.

Meadowsweet (*Filipendula ulmaria*)

Part used: Aerial parts

Actions: Antacid, anti-inflammatory, antirheumatic, astringent, carminative

Indications: Meadowsweet is one of the best digestive remedies available and as such will be indicated for many conditions, if they are approached holistically. It acts to protect and soothe the mucous membranes of the digestive tract, reducing excess acidity and easing nausea. It is used in the treatment of heartburn, hyperacidity, gastritis, and peptic ulceration. Its gentle astringency is useful in treating diarrhea in children. The presence of aspirin-like chemicals explains meadowsweet's action in reducing fever and relieving the pain of rheumatism in muscles and joints.

Dose: For an infusion, steep 1 to 2 teaspoons of the dried herb per cup of water and drink three times a day. For a tincture, take 1 to 2 milliliters three times a day.

Shepherd's Purse (*Capsella bursa-pastoris*)

Part used: Aerial parts

Actions: Anti-inflammatory, astringent, diuretic

Indications: As an astringent, shepherd's purse will prove effective in the treatment of diarrhea, wounds, and nosebleed. It is specific for stimulation of the menstrual process yet can also be used to reduce excess flow.

Dose: For an infusion, steep 1 to 2 teaspoons of the dried herb per cup of water and drink three times a day. For a tincture, take 1 to 2 milliliters three times a day.

Skullcap (*Scutellaria lateriflora*)

Part used: Aerial parts

Actions: Antispasmodic, hypotensive, nervine tonic

Indications: Skullcap is perhaps the most widely relevant nervine available to us. It relaxes states of nervous tension while at the same time it renews and revives the central nervous system. It has specific use in the treatment of hysterical states as well as epilepsy and other conditions involving seizures. It benefits all exhausted or depressed conditions and can be used with complete safety for easing premenstrual tension.

Dose: For an infusion, steep 1 to 2 teaspoons of the dried herb per cup of water and drink three times a day. For a tincture, take 2 to 4 milliliters three times a day.

St. John's Wort (*Hypericum perforatum*)

Part used: Flowering tops

Actions: Antidepressant, anti-inflammatory, antispasmodic, sedative, vulnerary

Indications: St. John's wort is one of Europe's best known wound-healing plants; it's used topically for this purpose. Used internally, it has a range of newly recognized uses for the nervous system, especially for the alleviation of stress and anxiety, but also for helping with depression.

Dose: For an infusion, steep 1 to 2 teaspoons of the dried herb per cup of water and drink twice a day. For topical use it is important to cover the area concerned, so use liberally. Also see the recipe for St. John's Wort Infused Oil on page 197. For a tincture, take 2.5 to 5 milliliters three times a day.

Thyme (*Thymus vulgaris*)

Part used: Leaves

Actions: Antimicrobial, antispasmodic, carminative, expectorant

Indications: The essential oil of thyme is strongly antiseptic, explaining many of the herb's uses. Thyme can be used externally as an ointment to heal wound infections but also internally for respiratory and digestive infections. It may be used as a gargle to ease laryngitis, tonsillitis, and sore throat. It is an excellent cough remedy, producing expectoration and reducing unnecessary spasm.

Dose: For an infusion, steep 1 to 2 teaspoons of the dried herb per cup of water and drink three times a day. For a tincture, take 1 to 2 milliliters three times a day.

Valerian (*Valeriana officinalis*)

Parts used: Rhizome and roots

Actions: Antispasmodic, carminative, hypnotic, hypotensive, nervine

Indications: Valerian is used to relieve tension and anxiety, whether the symptoms are purely psychological or physical in nature. It is a safe muscle relaxant and can be used to relieve muscle cramping, uterine cramps, and intestinal colic. It also helps with indigestion and nervous sleeplessness.

Dose: To be effective, valerian has to be used in sufficiently high dosage. For an infusion, steep 2 teaspoons of the dried root per cup of water and drink thirty minutes before bedtime. For a tincture, take 2.5 to 5 milliliters, and as much as 10 milliliters in some cases, thirty minutes before bedtime.

Witch Hazel (*Hamamelis virginiana*)

Parts used: Bark and leaves

Actions: Anti-inflammatory, astringent

Indications: Distilled witch hazel can be found in most households. It has a well-deserved reputation in the topical treatment of bruises, inflammation of the skin, and cuts and mild wounds with associated bleeding.

Dose: For an infusion, steep 1 teaspoon of the dried herb and apply topically as needed.

Yarrow (*Achillea millefolium*)

Part used: Aerial parts

Actions: Anti-inflammatory, antimicrobial, astringent, bitter, diaphoretic, diuretic, hypotensive

Indications: One of the best diaphoretic herbs, yarrow is a standard remedy for helping the body deal with fever. It lowers blood pressure by dilating peripheral blood vessels. Used externally, it aids in the healing of wounds.

Dose: For an infusion, steep 1 to 2 teaspoons of the dried herb per cup of water and drink three times a day.

The Medicine

The contribution herbalism can make in the trying times ahead is as much about pharmacy and medicine making as it is about the herbs themselves. In addition to knowing which plants are appropriate, the whole range of techniques inherent in traditional herbal medicine needs navigating. The core issue is making the therapeutic properties of the herb bioavailable to the body. Understanding the basic concepts of making herbal medicines is the practical basis of herbal health care, as often the nature of the medicine is as important as the herbs it might contain.

A characteristic of modern North American herbalism is the high level of skill and creativity evident in the herbal formulations created by herbalists, freeing the movement from dependency on what might be called "herb pharma"—the industry of commercial herbal products and the marketplace that supplies them.

This discussion is not about making medicines for the marketplace, but about basic herbal medicines for people to make and use in times of need. The techniques described here utilize common or easily learned skills to make simple yet effective medicines, with a long and solid history. Making these simple medicines from plants is no more challenging than cooking with plants! The simplicity of the techniques is a key factor that allows herbalism to be the people's medicine, avoiding the technological complexities of pseudopharma and the convoluted sophistications of the modern herb industry.

That said, simplicity of formulation and technique does not mean a medicine is less effective. The purpose of an herbal medicine is to make the therapeutic properties inherent within a plant available and active to the part of the body where they are needed. Success in this endeavor relies on two crucial issues: herbal chemistry and human physiology. Well-trained herbalists will know a great deal about these concepts, allowing creative formulation and targeted prescription, but even someone with just basic herbal literacy can make good simple medicine from plants.

The choice of technique is largely dictated by the chemistry of constituents considered responsible for therapeutic effects. For example, the active constituents of the relaxing, anxiety-reducing herb kava kava are the kavalactones, which are hardly soluble in water but readily soluble in alcohol. This means that a tea of kava kava would be pointless for delivery of the kavalactones. Alcohol- or even oil-based extracts would be the better choice.

Infusions

Infusions are the simplest, most common form of herbal medicine. These water-based extractions are appropriate for soft nonwoody plant material, such as leaves, flowers, and some stems. You can prepare an infusion from fresh or dried herbs, and in most cases it doesn't matter which one you use. If a formulation calls for one part of dried herb, it can be replaced with three parts of the fresh herb, the difference being due to the higher water content of the fresh herb.

To make an infusion:

1. Put 1 teaspoon of dried herb or 3 teaspoons of fresh herbs into a pot.
2. Pour 1 cup of boiling water over the herbs. Cover and let steep for ten to fifteen minutes.
3. Strain. Drink hot, cold, or iced.

To make larger quantities, use 1 ounce (30 grams) of dried herb for every 2 cups of water. If fresh herb is being used, remember that the material still contains meaningful amounts of water, so 1 part dried herb is usually considered to be equivalent to 3 parts fresh herb. Store a brewed infusion in the refrigerator.

Softer plant parts like leaves readily give up their constituents to heat. If you must make an infusion of sturdier plant parts, like bark, roots, or seeds, crush them first to break down some of the cell walls, thus making them more accessible to water. Be sure to cover an infusion while it is steeping to capture any aromatic volatile oils being released.

With herbs that are particularly sensitive to heat, with constituents that break down at high temperature, make a cold infusion. The proportion of herb to water is the same, but in this case the water is cold, not boiling, and the infusion should be left to steep for six to twelve hours in a well-sealed earthenware pot.

Decoctions

Decoctions, like infusions, are water-based herbal extracts, but they are appropriate for hard or woody plant material such as roots, bark, seeds, and nuts. The denser the plant material, the more energy is needed to extract its constituents into the water, explaining the value of decocting.

To make a decoction:

1. Put 1 teaspoon of dried herb or 3 teaspoons of fresh herb, cut into small pieces if needed, into a pot.
2. Add 1 cup water. Cover the pot. Bring to a boil, then reduce the heat and simmer for the amount of time specified for the mixture or specific herb, usually ten to fifteen minutes.
3. Strain while the tea is still hot, then drink.

As is the case for infusions, you can make and store larger quantities, using a ratio of 1 ounce (30 grams) of dried herb, or 3 ounces of fresh herb, for every 2 cups of water.

Tinctures

In general, alcohol and water together are a better solvent than water by itself for plant constituents, and at the same time they act as a preservative. Alcohol extracts are called tinctures. The method given here is a simple all-purpose one. When tinctures are prepared professionally, each herb has its own specific water-to-alcohol proportion, but such technicalities are unnecessary for general use. Be sure the alcohol is at least 60 proof (30 percent alcohol); this is about the weakest strength that still has a long-term preservative action. Vodka is generally a good choice.

To make an alcohol tincture:

1. Put 4 ounces (120 grams) of finely chopped or ground dried herb into a container that can be tightly closed. If you're using fresh herbs, use twice as much.
2. Pour 2 cups of vodka (30 alcohol/60 proof) over the herbs. Tightly seal the container.
3. Set the container in a warm place and let steep for two weeks. Shake it well twice every day.
4. Decant the liquid into a clean container. Pour the herb residue into a muslin cloth suspended over a bowl. Wring out all the liquid and add the rest of the tincture. The leftover plant matter makes excellent compost.
5. Pour the tincture into a dark bottle and seal tightly. Store in a cool, dark location, where it will keep indefinitely.

You can use the same tincturing process to prepare glycerin or vinegar extracts, simply substituting glycerin or vinegar for the alcohol.

Baths

Balneotherapy (from the Latin balneum, "bath") is the treatment of disease by bathing. Balneotherapy may involve hot or cold water, massage through moving water, relaxation, or stimulation. Often the best and most pleasant way of absorbing herbal compounds through the skin is by bathing in a full-body bath with 2 cups of an infusion or decoction added to the water. Alternatively, you can also take a foot or hand bath, in which case you would use the infusion or decoction in undiluted form.

Any herb that can be taken internally can be used in a bath. For example, for a bath that is relaxing and at the same time exquisitely scented, you could add an infusion of:

- Elder flower
- Lemon balm
- Linden
- Rosemary
- Rose petals

For a bath that will bring about a restful and healing sleep, add an infusion of one of the following:

- Chamomile
- Cramp bark
- Lavender
- Linden
- Valerian

Bear in mind that although valerian is very effective for promoting sleep, it has a strong aroma! For children with sleep problems or when babies are teething, try chamomile, linden, or red clover.

Oils

Many herbs are rich in essential oils. Some plants have essential oils that are volatile, which makes the plants aromatic, as is the case with mint. Others have essential oils that are not particularly volatile or aromatic, as is the case with St. John's wort. There are two methods of extracting essential oils: distillation and oil infusion.

Pure essential oils are extracted from an herb by a complex and careful process of distillation. These essential oils are best obtained from specialist suppliers who distill them as the basis for aromatherapy and as such take care that they are as pure as possible.

A much simpler method of extraction resembles cold water infusions. Instead of infusing the herb in water, you infuse it in an oil, obtaining a solution of the plant's essential oils in the oil base.

To make a simple infused herbal oil:

1. Chop the herb finely and put it in a clear glass container. Add enough oil to cover the plant matter. Almond oil is a good choice here. Other oils might also be used, but almond oil possesses a range of properties that make it especially useful in medicine making. It is highly emollient, which means that it helps balance the absorption of moisture and water loss, and it is a safe moisturizer that can be used on the body and face.
2. Place the container in the sun or in a warm place and let steep for two to three weeks. Shake the container daily.
3. Filter the infused oil into a dark glass container. Seal tightly and store in a cool, dark location, where it will keep for several months.

You can also more quickly extract a plant's constituents into an oil using the stovetop method: Combine the plant material and oil in a glass heatproof container, set the glass container in a pan of water, and warm over low heat for four hours.

🦌 St. John's Wort Infused Oil

St. John's wort's anti-inflammatory and wound-healing properties are unique and considered irreplaceable by most Western herbalists. The relevant constituents are especially soluble in oil, and so St. John's wort infused oil is a valuable topical application; it also blends readily with other topical healing herbs such as calendula.

Pick the flowering tops of St. John's wort when they have just opened. Crush the flowering tops in a teaspoonful of olive oil, then transfer the mixture to a glass container. Add enough oil to cover the plant matter and mix well. Place the container in the sun or in a warm place and let steep for three to six weeks. Shake the container daily. At the end of this time, the oil will be bright red.

Press the oil and herb mixture through a cloth (to filter the oil) into a clean container. Wrap the cloth up around the herb residue and wring out all the oil. Let the oil stand for a week. You will see some water in the liquid settling at the bottom. Decant just the oil from the top, not the watery liquid at the bottom, into a clean, dark glass container. Seal tightly and store in a cool, dark location, where it will keep for several months.

Ointments/Salves

Ointments, also known as salves, are semi-solid preparations that can be applied to the skin. Depending on the purpose for which they are designed, there are innumerable ways of making ointments; they can vary in texture from very greasy to a thick paste. Any herb can be used for making ointments, but particularly valuable for use in topical healing mixtures are arnica, calendula, chickweed, comfrey, goldenseal, plantain, slippery elm, thyme, and yarrow.

Aside from making simple herb teas, making a salve to heal damaged skin is perhaps the most important medicine-making technique to know. The following instructions for making a calendula ointment—a classic herbal preparation—can be used with any herb known to have topical healing properties.

🐾 Calendula Ointment

Extracting the healing properties of calendula requires a two-stage process. First the flowers are infused in an oil. Then the infused calendula oil is combined with a wax to create the ointment.

Stage 1: Calendula-Infused Oil
  1 cup dried calendula flowers
  8 ounces almond oil

Place the dried calendula in a glass, heat-proof container. Pour the almond oil over the flowers. Set the glass container in a pot of water, being careful not to let any water splash into the oil, and warm over low heat for four hours.

Let the infused oil cool until it is safe to handle. Strain the oil well.

Stage 2: Calendula Ointment
  4 ounces calendula infused oil
  ½ ounce beeswax, coarsely chopped
  20 drops lavender essential oil (optional)

Combine the calendula oil and beeswax in the top of a double boiler. Heat until the beeswax has melted and the mixture is blended. Remove from the heat. Stir in the lavender essential oil. Pour the mixture into tins or glass jars with lids. Let the ointment cool completely before placing lids on containers. Label the containers! Store in a cool, dry place, where the ointment will keep for two to three years.

Compress

A compress (technically a fomentation) is a simple way of applying a remedy to the skin and an excellent way to accelerate the healing process.

1. Soak a clean linen or cotton cloth in a hot herbal tea—as hot as can be tolerated—and apply it to the affected part of the body. Cover the soaked cloth with a towel to hold in the heat.
2. When the compress cools, replace it with another.

For a cold compress, use the same method but simply let the tea cool before soaking and applying.

Poultice

Similar to a compress, this more active application uses fresh or dried plant solids rather than a liquid form.

1. Mash or crush the plant material. Then either heat the mashed plant matter over boiling water in a double boiler or mix it with a small amount of boiling water to make a paste. If you're using powdered herb, mix it with boiling water to make a paste.
2. Apply the hot mashed herb—as hot as can be tolerated—directly to the skin, and hold it in place with gauze.

Some herbs, such as mustard, are especially stimulating. In this case, rather than applying them directly to the skin, sandwich them between two layers of cloth and then apply.

From Simples to Synergy:
Herbal Blends for Common Ailments

The simples (single herbs) discussed for the first aid kit (page 175) can be formulated into combinations that work synergistically, where the whole is more than the sum of the parts. This opens the possibility of focused blends that might be applicable in a variety of situations to address common symptoms and gently treat common pathologies. A blend formulated for use in alleviating the symptoms and discomfort of colds and the flu, for example, might also be broadly useful in fighting infection by supporting the body's immune response.

Following are a few examples of blends that would be broadly useful for community health care. It is in no way a comprehensive or definitive list, but indicative of the possibilities.

Cold Symptoms

The common cold is a viral infection of the upper respiratory system, but a number of infections and even allergies share a symptom picture that includes a runny nose, sore throat, and cough. Unfortunately, there is no universal cold cure; cold medicines, including herbal blends, are aimed simply at easing the symptoms. Regional cold care blends vary in the herbs they use, but a property they share is that of being diaphoretic—that is, they promote perspiration. This is a situation where the blend benefits from being formulated as a hot infusion of fresh or dried herbs. (See page 193 for infusion instructions.)

🐾 European Cold Care Blend

Elder flower
Peppermint
Yarrow

Blend equal parts of the herbs. Infuse the herb blend, using 1 to 2 teaspoons dried herb or 3 teaspoons fresh herb per cup of boiling water. Drink hot, often, until symptoms pass.

Influenza

Although often grouped with the common cold, influenza is a serious condition. The blend suggested here is not overtly antiviral but is intended to ease the discomforts, especially the aches and pains felt throughout the body. The intention is to ease the physical distress rather than kill viruses, and as such this blend may be used for other problems with such unpleasant symptoms. In addition to diaphoretics, the blend contains herbs that ease the muscular symptoms, of which boneset is the most important. Boneset has a strong bitter taste, which might stop some people from drinking a tea, so the blend is perhaps best formulated as a tincture (see page 195).

☙ Influenza Relief Blend

Boneset
Echinacea
Elder flower

Blend equal parts of the tincture of each herb. Adult dose: ½ teaspoon every three to four hours.

Insomnia

There can be no single blend here, because each person's needs are unique, and different herbs have different strengths and regionality—an important factor if the herbalist is relying on locally available stock. Mild effects can be expected from chamomile, lemon balm, linden blossom, and red clover; for children, these are the herbs to rely on. Effects can be noticeably stronger with motherwort, pulsatilla, and skullcap. The strongest effects would be seen with California poppy, hops, kava kava, passionflower, and valerian. *Caution:* Avoid the use of hops in depression.

☙ Sedative Blend

Kava kava
Passionflower
Valerian

Blend equal parts of the tincture of each herb. Adult dose: 1 to 2 teaspoons half an hour before bedtime.

Individualizing Blends

The blends presented here are easily tailored to address the specific issues an individual is managing. For example, with the sedative blend, selecting herbs that also address any health problems compounding the sleep difficulties obtains better results than simply a powerful hypnotic. The presence of heart palpitations might suggest the use of motherwort. Sleeplessness associated with indigestion would suggest the use of relaxing carminatives and bitters, as seen below.

₹ Blend for Sleeplessness with Indigestion

Lemon balm
Mugwort
Passionflower
Valerian

Blend equal parts of the tincture of the four herbs. Adult dose: 1 to 3 teaspoons half an hour before bedtime.

A tea of chamomile, linden, or lemon balm in the evening would also be helpful.

Muscular Tension and Rheumatism

The world abounds in plants that ease aches and pains. In this blend, meadowsweet is an anti-inflammatory that also settles gastric acidity, a common result of taking nonsteroidal anti-inflammatory drugs. Nettle is an alterative with a long history of use for rheumatic pain, and black cohosh—known as rheumatism root by the eclectics—is a uniquely effective anti-inflammatory in cases of rheumatism.

₹ Aches and Pains Blend

Black cohosh
Meadowsweet
Nettle

Blend equal parts of the tincture of each herb. Adult dose: 1 teaspoon three times a day.

Nausea

Nausea can result from a range of different issues, but alleviation of the unpleasant symptom can often be straightforward. There are many regional specifics, but an effective blend might be as follows.

❦ Nausea Relief Blend

Chamomile
Ginger
Peppermint

Blend equal parts of the tincture of each herb. Adult dose: ½ teaspoon three to five times a day.

Stress and Anxiety

Adaptogens, such as Siberian ginseng (eleuthero) and *Rhodiola* spp., specifically address the stress response. However, a limitation to their use is that they don't work rapidly, so relaxing nervines are essential, especially for acute situations. Herbs that can work quickly yet safely include gentle nervines such as lemon balm, linden, oats, and skullcap but also stronger ones such as passionflower, valerian, and wild lettuce. In the blend below, the focus is on herbs with a rapid experiential response, reducing psychological anxiety and the physical symptoms that might accompany it.

❦ Rapid Relaxation Blend

Milky oats
Skullcap
Valerian

Blend equal parts of the tincture of each herb. Adult dose: 1 teaspoon as needed.

It Takes a Village

Traditional herbal medicine can play a profoundly transformative role in how communities approach and facilitate health care in the face of the traumatic social and environmental challenges that predictably lie ahead. The heart of this contribution is the marriage of easily accessible health care with the agency of herbalists through community empowerment. Embedding the practice and knowledge of herbalism within a community offers its people the ability to define their own health care goals and act upon them. It is part of an ongoing process of supporting mutual respect, caring, and group participation, leading to people gaining control over their lives and democratic participation in the life of their community.

People cannot be empowered by others; they can only empower themselves. Community empowerment, therefore, is more than the involvement, participation, or engagement of communities. It implies community ownership and action that explicitly aims at social and political change. In a culture that is separated from the conscious embrace of nature, herbalism is inherently empowering.

There are a growing number of examples from around the country (and the world) of the ways in which herbalism embodies this bottom-up approach to community empowerment—examples that show why we might label this movement as people's herbalism.

Herbalista, based in Atlanta, Georgia, is a group of activist herbalists sponsoring health services and herbal education via creative programs designed to empower communities. They run a free clinic for the homeless and other vulnerable people, focusing on herb- and food-based therapy. They set up a bus as a mobile health care clinic. They established HerbCare Stations, providing free self-serve herbal health care products. All of these efforts bring health care services to traditionally underserved populations and empower people to care for themselves and their neighbors. Even more important, Herbalista uses the organization's own experience to actively promote other community-based ventures by herbalists worldwide, freely offering templates, instructions, workshops, feedback, and other support with the nuts and bolts of running a local grassroots project. (Facility with administrative practicalities does not always come easily to visionary herbalists!)

The Dublin Herb Bike is an example of the very practical results that come from the sort of support Herbalista provides. This organization, established with help from Herbalista, is a collective of herbalists who offer pop-up herbal wellness stations throughout Ireland, at shelters, community centers, and other places where there is need. Like Herbalista, the Dublin Herb Bike freely supports similar efforts by offering a template of instructions for its work (the *Herb Bike Manual*, easily found online), which provides basic protocols for mobile health care of all types.

The Botanical Bus, based in Sonoma County, California, is another example of people bringing herbalism to the people. The eponymous bus is a mobile health clinic offering bilingual, bicultural services to local farmworkers, primarily Latinx and Indigenous clients. The organization's staff includes promotoras, community members who receive specialized training so they can provide basic health education in the community without being a professional health care worker. The promotoras become a bridge between the diverse populations they serve and the health care system in general, taking on the role of advocate, educator, mentor, outreach worker, and interpreter. In addition, the organization offers Wellness Workshops, online and at family service centers, supporting community empowerment through herbal education and the exchange of locally made herbal medicines and recipes.

Emergent Herbalism

As herbalism reappears in the modern world, it is rapidly regaining respect as a source of unique knowledge that was ignored and almost lost by the mainstream. The rediscovery of herbalism runs the risk of being co-opted by some of the absurdities of the twenty-first century. The herb industry and the marketplace see healing plants as profit streams and the marketers dream of "low-hanging fruit." Similarly, the educational establishment is taking note of the demand from students for meaningful credit courses on herbalism.

This situation presents the modern herbalist with many challenges, especially how to fit into this brave new world without compromising the vision of herbalism as a holistic, empowering form of people's medicine.

One way for the herbalist to hold on to authenticity is to embrace and explore the tradition at the basis of their work and build conceptual and practical bridges from that solid foundation. An example of this can be seen in the work of Phyllis Light, an herbalist from Tennessee who grew up in the folk herbalism traditions of the Appalachian and Ozark mountains. Her training as a phytotherapist marries clinical science with respect for and deep knowledge of regional herbs and their preparation. Her herbal practice and educational work, focusing on local communities, are expressions of coevolution, seeing people's relationship with plants as food and medicine as going much deeper than the treatment of pathology, extending its reach into cultural, historical, economic, and even spiritual traditions within the region. This approach to herbalism recognizes the physical and psychological healing offered by herbs but also emphasizes the path of the herbalist as a catalyst for meaningful rituals and spiritual practice.

The herbal tradition once flourished among communities that were far more self-reliant than the complexities of modern life easily allow. Simple, place-based skills and knowledge (TEK) were shared via direct interactions with the village healer or community wise woman. From this perspective, herbalism is clearly a deeply nourishing and essential component of regenerative living. It's one we must learn, support, and transmit if humanity is to regenerate itself after the fall to come. The herbalist as activist must build the bridges of holistic health in the community, which in turn sows the seeds for the emergence of a truly resilient society, ready to cope with the uncertain future being faced.

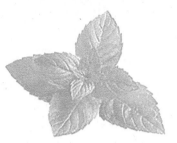

CONCLUSION

Herbalism in the Anthropocene

Herbalism is the medicine of belonging, an experience of the whole healing the part. In the face of humanity's blind abuse of nature and each other, we remember remedies that can help us survive the impact of our species' mistakes. It is an expression of real and practical links with nature, activating ecological relationships for healing. The simple act of taking herbal medicines creates a unique opportunity: a direct experience of belonging in the deepest sense. Herbalism abounds with opportunities to experience the healing presence of nature, whether in treating disease, growing medicine, or hugging a tree.

The simple skills and knowledge of traditional herbalism are uniquely suited to the challenges ahead. The skills of herbalism are basic, relevant, accessible, and low tech, and at the same time personally empowering. They will be an important part of any resilient response to the polycrisis, embodying herbalists' cumulative and evolving body of knowledge, practices, and beliefs about our relations with the ecosystem. Traditional herbalism offers ethical work in challenging times of social and cultural change.

Herbalism is as diverse as the people and the cultures they have created, and as we have seen, this diversity gifts humanity with locally relevant biocultural refugia of therapeutic plants and the memory of how to relate to them. This traditional ecological knowledge embodies the stewardship of biodiversity. It can strengthen the capacity of societies to deal with disturbances under conditions of uncertainty and change.

Human disconnection from the Earth is at the root of the polycrisis, and to address it we must shift our attitude of domination and reestablish our connection to the natural world. Herbalism can transform the way we view the world and be a foundational component of humanity reconciling with nature, our true family. In the coming years, we must focus on healing and reinvigorating fractured relationships, with each other, but especially in our relationship to the natural world.

The Taming Power of Small

Hexagram 9 in the *I Ching: Book of Changes* is "The Taming Power of Small," signifying a time when darkness has temporarily enveloped the light, representing the ability of the lesser to restrain the greater.

> The time is not yet for sweeping measures. Only through the small means can we exert any influence. However, we may be able, to a limited extent, to act as a restraining and subduing influence. To carry out our purpose we need firm determination within and gentleness and adaptability in external relations. Attempts made to press forward forcibly and change "the system" are doomed to failure. The entrenched "vested interest" are hindering meaningful change. (Wilhelm and Baynes 1950)

The work of all of who consider themselves activists is being degraded into the act of rearranging the deck chairs on the *Titanic*. Not because the work is useless or insignificant but because it will soon prove obsolete as we are overtaken by the tsunami of manifestations of the polycrisis.

The overarching issue is climate change. Whatever we may think, feel, project, or pray about it, strategies for changing it are now, as the English might say, like pissing in the wind. The central driver of it all is the amount of carbon in the air. Pandemic lockdowns rapidly reduced some signs of human damage to the planet. They were very welcome but very temporary cosmetic improvements. The beginning of any meaningful change is to change ourselves. And a crucial first step must be accepting what is.

Herbalism has often found itself on the wrong side of the establishment. The ebb and flow of its acceptance by the mainstream is an artifact of the changing fashions of the medical and legal elite in different cultures. However, the people of the world are very much in touch with the gifts of herbalism. The very existence of dissenters—whether herbalists, water activists, climate activists, or simple tree huggers—subverts and threatens the dominators. The corporatization of culture, and of the natural world, takes many forms, but most important is the devaluing and disempowerment of the non-corporate. Almost by definition, *non-corporate* here implies the herbalist.

We must be activists for many reasons, but in these times that try the soul we must be activists for the sake of our own humanity. The impulse to turn a blind eye is a very human response to the recognition that the future will be worse than the present, and especially that it's our fault. Something is terribly wrong, but a common response is to run and avoid, hiding in a mythical past. The deep crises we are in the midst of are bringing pain and suffering but also incredible opportunities for change. The world humanity has created might be ending, but that means things matter now more than ever.

It is time to challenge the idea of human supremacy on Earth.

Activism is more than what we do; it is also about who we are. It is about expressing regard, compassion, and love—for ourselves, for each other, and all the beings we share the world with. The implications of this concept are profound, but as Thich Nhat Hanh once said, "Real change will only happen when we fall in love with our planet."

Although we live in a time of pain and suffering, it is also a time that is rich in opportunities for change. The acceptance of *what is* changes perspectives; in the face of the existential threat, things matter more than ever. Choose to take action because it is how we get to truly live. Embrace the task of being authentically alive in a time of collapse. What might it take to be authentically alive in such a time?

On a deeply personal level, the despair must be faced and the choice made to take action, because in these times of crisis it is how we get to truly live. Seek out beauty, nurture it, and love it, finding your way to dance with the dark without falling in. Question everything as the profound transformations in mindsets and paradigms are underway.

First do no harm; then do the things that nurture the simple and be humble, showing kindness and generosity to others. Live creatively. Live ethically, taking responsibility for your life, your choices, and your actions in the world. There is social good in loving and caring for each other, whatever species we might be.

Recognize that we are deeply interconnected with other life forms and ecosystems. Value diversity in all forms, especially the gift of cultural and racial diversity. Protect biodiversity and build bridges. Reframe the relationships between humanity and nature, remembering that people thrive when life has conscious meaning and higher purpose.

Being in nature itself is potently healing. The return to bioregional and traditional practices around plants will restore the heart of herbalism and return us to true holism, where we acknowledge the wholeness of not only our own bodies but of the greater body of nature.

The Path of Conscious Simplicity

Our age of excess is destroying us, but there is a simple solution: herbalism as simplicity—the simple. What might be called the path of conscious simplicity reveals our sense of meaning and wonder, augmenting well-being and happiness for all.

Living on the Earth with other beings makes simplicity an ethical and ecological obligation. Taking simply what we need to sustain our life, living within ecological and planetary boundaries, leaves vital ecological space for other beings. Simplicity reduces humanity's ecological footprint. The consciousness that we are participants in the family of life on Earth, related and dependent on each other, naturally inspires compassion. When we see others as living members of our family rather than as objects or resources to be exploited, our first urge is to care, to share, to give.

Simplicity can be seen as a prerequisite for sustainability, helping to protect the planet and create ecological and economic justice. But living simply requires attention, awareness, and mindfulness. Optimism about technology assumes a future of sustained economic growth, eventually solving global poverty without destroying the ecosystems that sustain life. Such optimism is no longer justifiable. Response to the polycrisis requires a dramatic shift away from the economics of growth toward an economics beyond growth. It is time to degrow, to contract, downscaling both production and consumption.

Such degrowth could be achieved by planning and forward thinking, or it might be achieved through the polycrisis battling the marketplace. That is the radical implication of our global predicament that most people seem unwilling to acknowledge or accept. A necessary part of any transition to sustainability involves everyone adopting simpler lifestyles in terms of material and energy consumption. The move toward a just and sustainable economy that operates within safe limits depends on a vibrant, activist culture of voluntary simplicity—a culture of people choosing to restrain or reduce their material consumption, while at the same time seeking a higher quality of life.

Happiness cannot be bought, and well-being is not a commodity to be commercialized. Meaning and satisfaction in life come from being alive and not from having things; from relationships of care, compassion, and mutuality, not the violent appropriation of wealth. Choosing voluntary simplicity reduces our ecological footprint while increasing human well-being for all. Simplicity brings the awareness of "enoughness," of being content and satisfied with what one has or has achieved, without feeling the need for more. As Wendell Berry said, "To make a living is not to make a killing, it's to have enough" (Berry 2013). Appreciating life's abundance negates constantly striving for more. Enoughness can create the conditions needed for peace, both peace with nature and peace between people. Greed drives resource conflicts—wars with the Earth and wars against people. With the enoughness of simplicity, the conditions for peace with nature and peace between people can be created.

There is no easy way to navigate the planetary changes humanity has triggered. However, the planet is fine—if success is viewed as the saving of Earth, then success is assured, recognizing that the collective human species and the whole organism of Earth has self-healing, self-regenerating qualities.

The stark reality of the polycrisis calls for a reevaluation of plans and visions. Enough with obsessing about metric temperature measurements! Humanity has screwed up, and there is no stopping it. This perception of the likely future might seem depressingly dark, but only in light of the promised "bright" future of progress, with its enticements of development and continual "improvement." If this is actually seen as desirable, the future will be characterized by the hellish detritus of human failure.

That being said, in the new world we have entered, herbs, herbalism, and the herbalist have a major contribution to make to survival and resilience. This is the resilience of the human spirit expressed as the traditional ecological knowledge of herbalism—coevolutionary TEK.

The upwelling of herbal sensibilities we are seeing in people is one aspect of the collective consciousness's response to the polycrisis. The simple relationship of human and herb is an ecological reality gifted to us by evolution. The heart and soul of herbalism is the collective wisdom of herbalists, rich in traditional knowledge and skills, throughout time and around the world. It is blessed by generations of herbalists whose names and lives have been lost to history. Celebrate the unknown herbalist, all of our nameless sisters and brothers. Nothing is lost, only facts and figures, not the heart or soul or the herbs.

The best herbalism is local, reflecting the ecological family (community) that all people are part of. Plants are already everywhere we need them to be. From a simplistic perspective, it could be said that the supply chain is already growing in gardens, in the fields, even in the cracks in the sidewalk!

From Ariditas to Viriditas

Hildegard von Bingen's insight about the deeply ineffable quality of viriditas comes to the fore. Hildegard coined the word *viriditas*, or greening power, often described in the herbal community as the healing power of the divine in green things. Her vision sees the Creator bound to all creation, and especially humanity; "he showers upon it greening refreshment, the vitality to bear fruit" (Bingen 1983). Viriditas is immanent in all creation, but destruction of vibrant life leads to dryness and death, both physically and morally. Viriditas brings "lush greenness" to "shriveled and wilted" people and institutions, but its absence is the state of *ariditas*, or dryness, leading to the physical disease, which is the manifestation of such inhibition. The mindset exemplified by the dominant culture is a form of ariditas.

Viriditas is not only nature's divine healing power; it is a very personal expression of healing through the greening power of an herb, a quality Hildegard described as God's freshness. It is the energy that is always directed toward healing and wholeness. So green is not a mere color for Hildegard—it is an attitude and purposeful intent.

Plants play a profound role in human health and wholeness, and that healing relationship is one aspect of viriditas, but in terms of Hildegard's conceptualization, something much deeper is at play. Viriditas is the sap of herbalism worldwide. By "greening power," I interpret her to mean vital energy that is life, the spirit of the planet, the divine in a form that heals and transforms humanity.

Approaching herbalism from its array of diverse and divergent components illuminates a field of human endeavor that is a wonderful weaving of the miraculous and the mundane. It is a therapy that encompasses anthraquinone laxatives, the spiritual ecstasy of the Amazonian shaman, and the beauty of the flower. The limits to what might be called the path of the herbalist are only those imposed by parochial vision and a constipated imagination. Herbalism is part of the move away from anthropocentrism toward an affirmation of the wholeness of life.

It has been said that without vision, the people die. Without a personal vision, life becomes a slow process of degeneration and decay, and without some social vision, civilization rapidly disintegrates. Such a life-affirming vision is different from taking on a dogmatic belief system. It is an expression of meaning in an individual's life coming from their core. A green vision of humanity's place within the family of Gaia is illuminating our culture, and herbalism, with its reverence for life and bridging between plants and people, is at the heart of this transformation.

In light of all this, please accept this book as a contribution from a part to the whole, a perspective on herbalism whose simple ideas resonate with the needs of now. It has little to do with specific herbs or health care programs. It is an attempt at a bridge from the alienation deep within the psyche, the separation from the embrace of nature that plagues humanity. The healing offered so abundantly and freely by the plant kingdom is indeed a greening of the human condition, pointing to the reality of a new springtime. Humanity is awakening and finally finding its place within the biosphere, vibrantly alive, eyes wide open. With hearts that feel the love of the whales and the redwoods and minds revivified, we are filled with a vision of a healed world and ready for the challenges ahead.

Educational Resources

The herbal community of North America has dealt with the absence of mainstream pathways by creating a range of educational opportunities that are representative of the richness of modern herbalism. An excellent and regularly updated guide to suggested areas of study is offered by the American Herbalists Guild at AmericanHerbalistsGuild .com/herbal_education.

General Herbalism Programs

California School of Herbal Studies—David Hoffmann (CSHS.com)

Center for Herbal Studies—David Winston (HerbalStudies.net)

Columbines School of Botanical Studies—Howie Brounstein and Steven Yeager (BotanicalStudies.net)

East West School of Planetary Herbology—Michael and Lesley Tierra (PlanetHerbs.com)

Evergreen Herb Garden and School of Integrative Herbology—Candis Cantin (EvergreenHerbGarden.org)

Green Medicine Herb School—Kathi Keville (AHAHerb.com)

Herbal Transitions—Sharol Tilgner (HerbalTransitions.com)

Herbcraft—Jim McDonald (HerbCraft.org)

Northeast School of Botanical Medicine (7song.com)

Northwest School for Botanical Studies—Christa Sinadinos (HerbalEducation.net)

Sacred Plant Traditions Center for Herbal Studies—Kathleen Maier (SacredPlantTraditions.com)

The School of Natural Healing—David Christopher, MH (SNH.cc)

The Science & Art of Herbalism—Rosemary Gladstar (ScienceandArtOfHerbalism.com)

Southwest School of Botanical Medicine—Donna Chesner (SWSBM.com)

Vermont Center for Integrative Herbalism (VtHerbCenter.org)

Wise Woman Center—Susun Weed (SusunWeed.com)

Regional Focus

Appalachian Center for Natural Health—Appalachia (PhyllisDLight.com)

BotanoLogos School of Herbal Studies—Georgia (WildHealingHerbs.com)

Green Comfort School of Herbal Medicine—Virginia
(GreenComfortHerbSchool.com)

School of Ancestral Folk and Herbal Medicine—New Mexico
(NativeRootsSchool.com)

Strong Medical or Science Focus

Herbal medicine for women—Aviva Romm, MD (AvivaRomm.com/courses)

Foundations in herbal medicine—Tieraona Low Dog, MD (DrLowDog.com/
study-with-tieraona)

Foundations of herbalism—Christopher Hobbs, PhD, Lac
(FoundationsOfHerbalism.com)

Emergency Response and Herbal First Aid

Herbal Medics Academy (HerbalMedics.academy), a branch of the Human
Path school, founded by Sam Coffman. The academy's focus is on botanical medicine in the context of emergency response and wilderness first aid.

Veterinary Herbal Education

Purple Moon Herbs & Studies (PurpleMoonHerbStudies.com)

References

Abdel-Lateif, Khalid, Didier Bogusz, and Valérie Hocher. 2012. "The Role of Flavonoids in the Establishment of Plant Roots Endosymbioses with Arbuscular Mycorrhiza Fungi, Rhizobia and Frankia Bacteria." *Plant Signaling and Behavior* 7 (6): 636–41.

Aboulghazi, Abderrazak, Soumaya Touzani, Mouhcine Fadil, and Badiaa Lyoussi. 2022. "Physicochemical Characterization and *In Vitro* Evaluation of the Antioxidant and Anticandidal Activities of Moroccan Propolis." *Veterinary World* 15 (2): 341.

Allaby, Robin G., Logan Kistler, Rafal M. Gutaker, Roselyn Ware, James L. Kitchen, Oliver Smith, and Andrew C. Clarke. 2015. "Archaeogenomic Insights into the Adaptation of Plants to the Human Environment: Pushing Plant–Hominin Co-evolution Back to the Pliocene." *Journal of Human Evolution* 79: 150–57.

Allkin, Bob. 2017. "Useful Plants—Medicines: At Least 28,187 Plant Species Are Currently Recorded as Being of Medicinal Use." In *State of the World's Plants*, edited by Kathy J. Willis. London: Royal Botanic Gardens, Kew.

American Museum of Natural History. n.d. "What Is Biodiversity?" American Museum of Natural History Center for Biodiversity & Conservation website. Accessed September 26, 2023.

Antonelli, Michele, Davide Donelli, Grazia Barbieri, Marco Valussi, Valentina Maggini, and Fabio Firenzuoli. 2020. "Forest Volatile Organic Compounds and Their Effects on Human Health: A State-of-the-Art Review." *International Journal of Environmental Research and Public Health* 17 (18): 6506.

Applequist, W. L., J. A. Brinckmann, A. B. Cunningham, R. E. Hart, M. Heinrich, D. R. Katerere, and T. van Andel. 2020. "Scientists' Warning on Climate Change and Medicinal Plants." *Planta Medica* 86 (1): 10–18.

Bannister, C. A., S. E. Holden, S. Jenkins-Jones, et al. 2014. "Can People with Type 2 Diabetes Live Longer than Those Without? A Comparison of Mortality in People Initiated with Metformin or Sulphonylurea Monotherapy and Matched, Non-diabetic Controls." *Diabetes, Obesity and Metabolism* 16 (11): 1165–73.

Barbosa, A. P. 2014. "An Overview on the Biological and Pharmacological Activities of Saponins." *International Journal of Pharmacy and Pharmaceutical Sciences* 6 (8): 47–50.

Barth, F., and M. Rinaldi-Carmona. 1999. "The Development of Cannabinoid Antagonists." *Current Medicinal Chemistry* 6: 745–56.

Barthel, S., C. L. Crumley, and U. Svedin. 2013. "Biocultural Refugia: Combating the Erosion of Diversity in Landscapes of Food Production." *Ecology and Society* 18 (4): 71.

BBC News. 2005. "Port Talbot Tops Pollution Chart." BBC News webpage. Last updated February 28, 2005.

Beck, Andrew H. 2004. "The Flexner Report and the Standardization of American Medical Education." *JAMA* 291 (17): 2139–40.

Berry, Wendell. 2013. "Segment: Wendell Berry on His Hopes for Humanity." Interview by Bill Moyers on *Moyers & Company*, October 4, 2013.

Bingen, Hildegard von. 1983. *Meditations with Hildegard of Bingen*. Edited by Gabriele Uhlein. Rochester, Vt.: Bear & Company.

Blumenthal, Mark. 2000. *Herbal Medicine: Expanded Commission E Monographs*. 1st ed. Newton, Mass.: Integrative Medicine Communications.

Bonfante, Paola, and Andrea Genre. 2010. "Mechanisms Underlying Beneficial Plant-Fungus Interactions in Mycorrhizal Symbiosis." *Nature Communications* 1: 48.

Bostrom, N. 2013. "Existential Risk Prevention as Global Priority." *Global Policy* 4 (1): 15–31.

Brundrett, Mark C. 2002. "Coevolution of Roots and Mycorrhizas of Land Plants." *New Phytologist* 154 (2): 275–304.

Butler, Mark S., Avril A. B. Robertson, and Matthew A. Cooper. 2014. "Natural Product and Natural Product Derived Drugs in Clinical Trials." *Natural Product Reports* 31 (11): 1612–61.

Carlson, E. E. 2010. "Natural Products as Chemical Probes." *ACS Chemical Biology* 5 (7): 639–53.

Casas, Ana I., Ahmed A. Hassan, Simon J. Larsen, et al. 2019. "From Single Drug Targets to Synergistic Network Pharmacology in Ischemic Stroke." *Proceedings of the National Academy of Sciences* 116 (14): 7129–36.

Chen, Chun, Qishi Song, Magali Proffit, Jean-Marie Bessière, Zong-Bo Li, and Martine Hossaert-McKey. 2009. "Private Channel: A Single Unusual Compound Assures Specific Pollinator Attraction in Ficus semicordata." *Functional Ecology* 23 (5): 941–50.

Coffman, Sam. 2021. *Herbal Medic: A Green Beret's Guide to Emergency Medical Preparedness and Natural First Aid*. North Adams, Mass.: Storey Publishing.

Cohen, Deatra, and Adam Siegel. 2021. *Ashkenazi Herbalism: Rediscovering the Herbal Traditions of Eastern European Jews.* Berkeley, Calif.: North Atlantic Books.

Commoner, Barry. 1971. *The Closing Circle.* New York: Alfred A. Knopf.

Cunsolo, A., S. L. Harper, K. Minor, K. Hayes, K. G. Williams, and C. Howard. 2020. "Ecological Grief and Anxiety: The Start of a Healthy Response to Climate Change?" *The Lancet Planetary Health* 4 (7): e261–e263.

Davis, G. F., and S. Kim. 2015. "Financialization of the Economy." *Annual Review of Sociology* 41 (1): 203–21.

de Carvalho, O., Jr., S. F. Ferrari, and K. B. Strier. 2004. "Diet of a Muriqui Group (Brachyteles arachnoides) in Continuous Primary Forest." *Primates* 45 (3): 201–4.

de Macedo, Lucas Malvezzi, Érica Mendes Dos Santos, Lucas Militão, Louise Lacalendola Tundisi, Janaína Artem Ataide, Eliana Barbosa Souto, and Priscila Gava Mazzola. 2020. "Rosemary (*Rosmarinus officinalis* L., syn *Salvia rosmarinus* Spenn.) and Its Topical Applications: A Review." *Plants* (Basel) 9 (5): 651.

Department of the Air Force, Office of the Assistant Secretary for Energy, Installations, and Environment. 2022. *Department of the Air Force Climate Action Plan.* Washington, DC: October 2022.

Devitt, Elizabeth. 2015. "The Muriqui: Brazil's Critically Endangered 'Hippie Monkey' Hangs Tough." Mongabay Series: Almost Famous Animals, October 12, 2015.

De Vos, Jurriaan M., Lucas N. Joppa, John L. Gittleman, Patrick R. Stephens, and Stuart L. Pimm. 2015. "Estimating the Normal Background Rate of Species Extinction." *Conservation Biology* 29 (2): 452–62.

Dias, Daniel A., Sylvia Urban, and Ute Roessner. 2012. "A Historical Overview of Natural Products in Drug Discovery." *Metabolites* 16 (2): 303–36.

Dixon, Neil, Lu Shin Wong, Torsten H. Geerlings, and Jason Micklefield. 2007. "Cellular Targets of Natural Products." *Natural Product Reports* 24 (6): 1288–1310.

Dixon, Richard A., and Dieter Strack. 2003. "Phytochemistry Meets Genome Analysis, and Beyond." *Phytochemistry* 62 (6): 815–16.

DOD News. 2015. "DoD Releases Report on Security Implications of Climate Change." U.S. Department of Defense website, July 29, 2015.

Dong, Xiaoxv, Jing Fu, Xingbin Yin, Sali Cao, Xuechun Li, Longfei Lin, et al. 2016. "Emodin: A Review of Its Pharmacology, Toxicity and Pharmacokinetics." *Phytotherapy Research* 30 (8): 1207–18.

Drinkwater, N. R., E. C. Miller, J. A. Miller, and H. C. Pitot. 1976. "Hepatocarcinogenicity of Estragole (1-allyl-4-methoxybenzene) and 1'-hydroxyestragole in the Mouse and Mutagenicity of 1'-acetoxyestragole in Bacteria." *Journal of National Cancer Institute* 57 (6): 1323–31.

Duarte Santos, Filipe. 2021. "Anthropocene, Technosphere, Biosphere, and the Contemporary Utopias." In *Time, Progress, Growth and Technology*, 381–542. Cham, Switzerland: Springer.

Ellis, E. C., and P. K. Haff. 2009. "Earth Science in the Anthropocene: New Epoch, New Paradigm, New Responsibilities." *Eos* 90 (49): 473.

EMA (European Medicines Agency). 2023. "Public Statement on the Use of Herbal Medicinal Products Containing Estragole." EMA/HMPC/137212/2005 Rev 1 Corr 1. Committee on Herbal Medicinal Products (HMPC). May 12, 2023.

FAO and UNEP. 2020. The State of the World's Forests 2020. Forests, Biodiversity and People. Rome: Food and Agriculture Organization of the United Nations.

Ferreira, Jorge F. S., Devanand L. Luthria, Tomikazu Sasaki, and Arne Heyerick. 2010. "Flavonoids from Artemisia annua L. as Antioxidants and Their Potential Synergism with Artemisinin against Malaria and Cancer." *Molecules* 15 (5): 3135–70.

Fisch, M. H. 1945. "Pharmacopoeia Londinensis of 1618, Reproduced in Facsimile, with a Historical Introduction." *Bulletin of the Medical Library Association* 33 (4): 541–42.

Foster, Steven. 1993. *Herbal Renaissance: Growing, Using & Understanding Herbs in the Modern World*. Kaysville, Utah: Gibbs Smith.

Fowler, Andrew, Yianna Koutsioni, and Volker Sommer. 2007. "Leaf-Swallowing in Nigerian Chimpanzees: Evidence for Assumed Self-Medication." *Primates* 48 (1): 73–76.

Frey, E. F. 1985. "The Earliest Medical Texts." *Clio Medica* 20 (1–4): 79–90.

Gershenzon, Jonathan, and Natalia Dudareva. 2007. "The Function of Terpene Natural Products in the Natural World." *Nature Chemical Biology* 3 (7): 408–14.

Gladstar, Rosemary. n.d. "Growing Awareness with Botanical Sanctuaries." Blog post for Rosemary Gladstar's The Science & Art of Herbalism. Accessed October 18, 2023.

Gori, L., E. Gallo, V. Mascherini, A. Mugelli, A. Vannacci, and F. Firenzuoli. 2012. "Can Estragole in Fennel Seed Decoctions Really Be Considered a Danger for Human Health? A Fennel Safety Update." *Evidence-Based Complementary and Alternative Medicine* 2012: 860542.

Greene, A. M., P. Panyadee, A. Inta, and M. A. Huffman. 2020. "Asian Elephant Self-Medication as a Source of Ethnoveterinary Knowledge among Karen Mahouts in Northern Thailand." *Journal of Ethnopharmacology* 259: 112823.

Groening, G., and J. Wolschke-Bulmahn. 1992. "Some Notes on the Mania for Native Plants in Germany." *Landscape Journal* 11 (2): 116–26.

Guenthner T. M., and G. Luo G. 2001. "Investigation of the Role of the

2',3'-epoxidation Pathway in the Bioactivation and Genotoxicity of Dietary Allylbenzene Analogs." *Toxicology* 160: 47–58.

Gwinner, Helga. 2012. "Male European Starlings Use Odorous Herbs as Nest Material to Attract Females and Benefit Nestlings." In *Chemical Signals in Vertebrates* 12, 353–62. New York: Springer.

Hale, T. W., and H. E. Rowe. 2016. *Medications and Mothers' Milk 2017.* Springer Publishing Company.

Hallmann, Caspar A., Martin Sorg, Eelke Jongejans, Henk Siepel, Nick Hofland, et al. 2017. "More Than 75 Percent Decline over 27 Years in Total Flying Insect Biomass in Protected Areas." *PloS One* 12 (10): e0185809.

Hammerbacher, Almuth, Teresa A. Coutinho, and Jonathan Gershenzon. 2019. "Roles of Plant Volatiles in Defence against Microbial Pathogens and Microbial Exploitation of Volatiles." *Plant, Cell & Environment* 42 (10): 2827–43.

Harborne, J. B. 1993. *Introduction to Ecological Biochemistry.* 4th ed. London: Elsevier.

Hardy, Karen. 2019. "Paleomedicine and the Use of Plant Secondary Compounds in the Paleolithic and Early Neolithic." *Evolutionary Anthropology: Issues, News, and Reviews* 28 (2): 60–71.

———. 2021. "Paleomedicine and the Evolutionary Context of Medicinal Plant Use." *Revista Brasileira de Farmacognosia* 31 (1): 1–15.

Hartz, Kara E. Huff, Thomas Rosenørn, Shaun R. Ferchak, Timothy Michael Raymond, Merete Bilde, Neil M. Donahue, and Spyros N. Pandis. 2005. "Cloud Condensation Nuclei Activation of Monoterpene and Sesquiterpene Secondary Organic Aerosol." *Journal of Geophysical Research: Atmospheres* 110 (14).

Hassan, Samira, and Ulrike Mathesius. 2012. "The Role of Flavonoids in Root–Rhizosphere Signalling: Opportunities and Challenges for Improving Plant–Microbe Interactions." *Journal of Experimental Botany* 63 (9): 3429–44.

He, M., M. Halima, Y. Xie, M. J. Schaaf, A. H. Meijer, and M. Wang. 2020. "Ginsenoside Rg1 Acts as a Selective Glucocorticoid Receptor Agonist with Anti-inflammatory Action without Affecting Tissue Regeneration in Zebrafish Larvae." *Cells* 9 (5): 1107.

Heckman, D. S., D. M. Geiser, B. R. Eidell, R. L. Stauffer, N. L. Kardos, and S. B. Hedges. 2018. "Molecular Evidence for the Early Colonization of Land by Fungi and Plants." *Science* 293 (5532): 1129–33.

Hermann, C. 2021. *The Critique of Commodification: Contours of a Post-capitalist Society.* New York: Oxford University Press.

Hill, John. 1756. *The British Herbal: An History of Plants and Trees, Natives of Britain, Cultivated for Use, or Raised for Beauty.* London: Printed for

T. Osborne, J. Shipton, J. Hodges, J. Newbery, B. Collins, S. Crowder, and H. Woodgate.

Hillard, C. J. 2015. "Endocannabinoids and the Endocrine System in Health and Disease." *Handbook of Experimental Pharmacology* 231: 317–39.

Hills, J. M., and P. I. Aaronson. 1991. "The Mechanism of Action of Peppermint Oil on Gastrointestinal Smooth Muscle." *Gastroenterology* 101 (1): 55–65.

Hinsley, A., E. J. Milner-Gulland, R. Cooney et al. 2020. "Building Sustainability into the Belt and Road Initiative's Traditional Chinese Medicine Trade." *Nature Sustainability* 3: 96–100.

Hoffmann, David. 1998. *The Herbal Handbook: A User's Guide to Medical Herbalism*. Rochester, Vt.: Healing Arts Press.

———. 2003. *Medical Herbalism: The Science and Practice of Herbal Medicine*. Rochester, Vt.: Healing Arts Press.

Honda, K. 1990. "Identification of Host-Plant Chemicals Stimulating Oviposition by Swallowtail Butterfly, Papilio protenor." *Journal of Chemical Ecology* 16 (2): 325–37.

Hong, Jiyong. 2011. "Role of Natural Product Diversity in Chemical Biology." *Current Opinion in Chemical Biology* 15 (3): 350–54.

Hool, Richard Lawrence. 1922. *Common Plants and Their Uses in Medicine*. Lancashire, U.K.: National Association of Medical Herbalists.

Huffman, Michael A. 2001. "Self-Medicative Behavior in the African Great Apes." *BioScience* 51 (8): 651–61.

———. 2022. "Folklore, Animal Self-Medication, and Phytotherapy: Something Old, Something New, Something Borrowed, Some Things True." *Planta Medica* 88 (3-04): 187–99.

Idowu, Samuel O., Nicholas Capaldi, Liangrong Zu, and Ananda Das Gupta, eds. 2013. *Encyclopedia of Corporate Social Responsibility*, vol. 21. Berlin: Springer.

Janeczko, A., and A. Skoczowski. 2005. "Mammalian Sex Hormones in Plants." *Folia Histochemica et Cytobiologica* 43 (2): 71–79.

Jenke-Kodama, Holger, Rolf Müller, and Elke Dittmann. 2008. "Evolutionary Mechanisms Underlying Secondary Metabolite Diversity." *Progress in Drug Research* 65: 119, 121–40.

Jenkins, M., A. Timoshyna, and M. Cornthwaite. 2018. *Wild at Home: Exploring the Global Harvest, Trade and Use of Wild Plant Ingredients*. Cambridge, U.K.: TRAFFIC International.

Junio, Hiyas A., Arlene A. Sy-Cordero, Keivan A. Ettefagh, Johnna T. Burns, Kathryn T. Micko, Tyler N. Graf, et al. 2011. "Synergy Directed Fractionation of Botanical Medicines: A Case Study with Goldenseal (*Hydrastis canadensis*)." *Journal of Natural Products* 74 (7): 1621–29.

Kelly, M. 2001. *The Divine Right of Capital: Dethroning the Corporate Aristocracy.* Berrett-Koehler Publishers.

Kemp, Luke. 2019. "The Lifespans of Ancient Civilisations." BBC Future (online), February 19, 2019.

Kennedy, D. O., and E. L. Wightman. 2011. "Herbal Extracts and Phytochemicals: Plant Secondary Metabolites and the Enhancement of Human Brain Function." *Advances in Nutrition* 2 (1): 32–50.

Kessler, A., and I. T. Baldwin. 2001. "Defensive Function of Herbivore Induced Plant Volatile Emissions in Nature." *Science* 291: 2141–44.

Kligler, B., and S. Chaudhary. 2007. "Peppermint Oil." *American Family Physician* 75 (7): 1027–30.

Kramer, Heinrich, and James Sprenger. 2007. *The Malleus Maleficarum.* New York: Cosimo.

Kremers, Edward, Glenn Sonnedecker, and George Urdang. 1986. *Kremers and Urdang's History of Pharmacy.* 4th ed. Madison, Wisc.: American Institute of the History of Pharmacy.

Kuhn, Thomas S. 2012. *The Structure of Scientific Revolutions.* 50th anniversary ed. Chicago: University of Chicago.

Lambrechts, M. M., and A. D. Santos. 2000. "Aromatic Herbs in Corsican Blue Tit Nests: The Potpourri Hypothesis." *Acta Oecologica* 21 (3): 175–78.

Lanfranco, Luisa, Paola Bonfante, and Andrea Genre. 2016. "The Mutualistic Interaction between Plants and Arbuscular Mycorrhizal Fungi." *Microbiology Spectrum* 4 (6).

Larsen, B. B., E. C. Miller, M. K. Rhodes, and J. J. Wiens. 2017. "Inordinate Fondness Multiplied and Redistributed: The Number of Species on Earth and the New Pie of Life." *Quarterly Review of Biology* 92 (3): 229–65.

Li, Q. 2010. "Effect of Forest Bathing Trips on Human Immune Function." *Environmental Health and Preventive Medicine* 15 (1): 9–17.

Liao, W., Q. Jin, J. Liu, et al. 2021. "Mahuang Decoction Antagonizes Acute Liver Failure via Modulating Tricarboxylic Acid Cycle and Amino Acids Metabolism." *Frontiers in Pharmacology* 12: 599180.

Liu, Ping, Songlin Liu, Daizhi Tian, and Ping Wang. 2012. "The Applications and Obstacles of Metabonomics in Traditional Chinese Medicine." *Evidence-Based Complementary and Alternative Medicine* 2012: 945824.

Lopresti, A. L. 2017. "Salvia (Sage): A Review of Its Potential Cognitive-Enhancing and Protective Effects." *Drugs in R&D* 17 (1): 53–64.

Loreto, Francesco, Francesca Bagnoli, Carlo Calfapietra, et al. 2013. "Isoprenoid Emission in Hygrophyte and Xerophyte European Woody Flora: Ecological and Evolutionary Implications." *Global Ecology and Biogeography* 23 (3): 334–45.

Luginbuehl, Leonie H., and Giles E. D. Oldroyd. 2017. "Understanding the Arbuscule at the Heart of Endomycorrhizal Symbioses in Plants." *Current Biology* 27 (17): 952–63.

Mackay, C. 1841. *Memoirs of Extraordinary Popular Delusions and the Madness of Crowds.* Vol. 1. London: George Routledge and Sons.

Maggi, F., and F. H. Tang. 2021. "Estimated Decline in Global Earthworm Population Size Caused by Pesticide Residue in Soil." *Soil Security* 5: 100014.

Mailett, Fabienne, Véréna Poinsot, Olivier André, Virginie Puech-Pagès, Alexandra Haouy, Monique Gueunier, Laurence Cromer, Delphine Giraudet, Damien Formey, Andreas Niebel, Eduardo Andres Martinez, Hugues Driguez, Guillaume Bécard, and Jean Dénarié. 2011. "Fungal Lipochito-oligosaccharide Symbiotic Signals in Arbuscular Mycorrhiza." *Nature* 469: 58–63.

Mao, Wanying, Medard Adu, Ejemai Eboreime, et al. 2022. "Post-Traumatic Stress Disorder, Major Depressive Disorder, and Wildfires: A Fifth-Year Postdisaster Evaluation among Residents of Fort McMurray." *International Journal of Environmental Research and Public Health* 19 (15): 9759.

Margetts, G., S. Kleidonas, N. S. Zaibi, M. S. Zaibi, and K. D. Edwards. 2022. "Evidence for Anti-inflammatory Effects and Modulation of Neurotransmitter Metabolism by *Salvia officinalis* L." *BMC Complementary Medicine and Therapies* 22 (1): 131.

Margulis, Lynn, and Dorion Sagan. 2002. *Acquiring Genomes: A Theory of the Origin of Species.* Basic Books.

Micale, V., and F. Drago. 2018. "Endocannabinoid System, Stress and HPA Axis." *European Journal of Pharmacology* 834: 230–39.

Miranda Chaves, Sérgio Augusto de, and Karl J. Reinhard. 2006, "Critical Analysis of Coprolite Evidence of Medicinal Plant Use, Piauí, Brazil." *Palaeogeography, Palaeoclimatology, Palaeoecology* 237 (1): 110-18.

Mora, Camilo, Derek P. Tittensor, Sina Adl, Alastair G. B. Simpson, and Boris Worm. 2011. "How Many Species Are There on Earth and in the Ocean?" *PLoS biology* 9 (8): e1001127.

Moreira, F. A., and J. A. S. Crippa. 2009. "The Psychiatric Side-Effects of Rimonabant." *Brazilian Journal of Psychiatry* 31: 145–53.

Morrogh-Bernard, H. C., I. Foitová, Z. Yeen, P. Wilkin, R. de Martin, L. Rárová, K. Doležal, W. Nurcahyo, and M. Olšanský. 2017. "Self-Medication by Orang-utans (*Pongo pygmaeus*) Using Bioactive Properties of Dracaena cantleyi." *Scientific Reports* 7 (1): 1–7.

Nelsen, Jamie, Catherine Ulbricht, Ernie Paul Barrette, David Sollars, Candy Tsourounis, Adrianne Rogers, Samuel Basch, Sadaf Hashmi, Steve Bent, and Ethan Basch. 2002. "Red Clover (Trifolium pratense) Monograph: A Clinical

Decision Support Tool." *Journal of Herbal Pharmacotherapy* 2 (3): 49–72.

Newman, David J., and Gordon M. Cragg. 2016. "Natural Products as Sources of New Drugs from 1981 to 2014." *Journal of Natural Products* 79 (3): 629–61.

Ninkuu, Vincent, Lin Zhang, Jianpei Yan, Zhenchao Fu, Tengfeng Yang, and Hongmei Zeng. 2021. "Biochemistry of Terpenes and Recent Advances in Plant Protection." *International Journal of Molecular Sciences* 22 (11): 5710.

Nishida, Ritsuo. 2014. "Chemical Ecology of Insect–Plant Interactions: Ecological Significance of Plant Secondary Metabolites." *Bioscience, Biotechnology, and Biochemistry* 78 (1): 1–13.

Otto, Eduard. 1993. "Das Dresdner Experiment: Naturheilmethoden sollten überprüft werden." *Deutsches Ärzteblatt* 90: 948–51.

Pan, F. 2011. "Doadi Medicinal Material Is the Essence of Chinese Medicine—A Review of the 390th Session of Xiangshan Science Conference." *Science Times*, February 28, 2011, Beijing, China.

Pan, S. Y., G. Litscher, S. H. Gao, S. F. Zhou, Z. L. Yu, H. Q. Chen, S. F. Zhang, M. K. Tang, J. N. Sun, and K. M. Ko. 2014. "Historical Perspective of Traditional Indigenous Medical Practices: The Current Renaissance and Conservation of Herbal Resources." Evidence-Based Complementary and Alternative Medicine 2014: 525340.

Panossian, Alexander, Marina Hambardzumyan, Areg Hovhanissyan, and Georg Wikman. 2007. "The Adaptogens Rhodiola and Schizandra Modify the Response to Immobilization Stress in Rabbits by Suppressing the Increase of Phosphorylated Stress-Activated Protein Kinase, Nitric Oxide and Cortisol." *Drug Target Insights* 2: 39–54.

Panossian, Alexander, Rebecca Hamm, Onat Kadioglu, Georg Wikman, and Thomas Efferth. 2013. "Synergy and Antagonism of Active Constituents of ADAPT-232 on Transcriptional Level of Metabolic Regulation of Isolated Neuroglial Cells." *Frontiers in Neuroscience* 7: 16.

Parejo I., F. Viladomat, J. Bastida, A. Rosas-Romero, N. Flerlage, J. Burillo, and C. Codina. 2002. "Comparison between the Radical Scavenging Activity and Antioxidant Activity of Six Distilled and Nondistilled Mediterranean Herbs and Aromatic Plants." *Journal of Agricultural and Food Chemistry* 50: 6882–90.

Pearce, Richard B. 2017. "Joe Pye, Joe Pye's Law, and Joe-Pye-Weed: The History and Eponymy of the Common Name Joe-Pye-Weed for Eutrochium Species (Asteraceae)." *The Great Lakes Botanist* 56: 177–200.

Perkins, M. W. 1618. *A Discourse of the Damned Art of Witchcraft; So Farre Forth as It Is Revealed in the Scriptures, and Manifest by True Experience.* Cambridge: Cantrelle Legge, printer to the University of Cambridge.

Persons, W. S. 1994. *American Ginseng: Green Gold.* Rev. ed. Asheville, N.C.: Bright Mountain Books.

Pertwee, Roger G. 2006. "Cannabinoid Pharmacology: The First 66 Years." *British Journal of Pharmacology* 147 (S1): 163–71.

Phillips D. H., J. A. Miller, E. C. Miller, and B. Adams. 1981. "Structures of the DNA Adducts Formed in Mouse Liver after Administration of the Proximate Hepatocarcinogen 1'-hydroxyestragole." *Cancer Research* 44 (41): 176–86.

Prattichizzo, Francesco, Angelica Giuliani, et al. 2018. "Pleiotropic Effects of Metformin: Shaping the Microbiome to Manage Type 2 Diabetes and Postpone Ageing." *Ageing Research Reviews* 48: 87–98.

Rai, Amit, Kazuki Saito, and Mami Yamazaki. 2017. "Integrated Omics Analysis of Specialized Metabolism in Medicinal Plants." *The Plant Journal* 90 (4): 764–87.

Remy, W., T. N. Taylor, H. Hass, and H. Kerp. 1994. "Four Hundred-Million-Year-Old Vesicular Arbuscular Mycorrhizae." *Proceedings of the National Academy of Sciences* 91 (25): 11841–43.

Reuss, Walter. 2013. *Hagers Handbuch der Pharmazeutischen Praxis*. Vol. 1. Berlin: Springer.

Reyes-García, Victoria, Jaime Paneque-Gálvez, Ana C. Luz, Maximillien Gueze, Manuel J. Macía, Martí Orta-Martínez, and Joan Pino. 2014. "Cultural Change and Traditional Ecological Knowledge. An Empirical Analysis from the Tsimane' in the Bolivian Amazon." *Human Organization* 73 (2): 162–73.

Rhodes, Marissa. 2020. "Both Man and Witch: Uncovering the Invisible History of Male Witches." *Dig: A History Podcast*, September, 13, 2020.

Ripple, W. J., C. Wolf, J. W. Gregg, et al. 2022. "World Scientists' Warning of a Climate Emergency 2022." *BioScience* 72 (12): 1149–55.

Rogers, Kara, ed. 2011. *Medicine and Healers through History*. New York: Britannica Educational Publishing.

Russo, Gian Luigi, Maria Russo, and Carmela Spagnuolo. 2014. "The Pleiotropic Flavonoid Quercetin: From Its Metabolism to the Inhibition of Protein Kinases in Chronic Lymphocytic Leukemia." *Food & Function* 5 (10): 2393-240i.

Russo, Gian Luigi, Maria Russo, Carmela Spagnuolo, Idolo Tedesco, Stefania Bilotto, Roberta Iannitti, and Rosanna Palumbo. 2014. "Quercetin: A Pleiotropic Kinase Inhibitor against Cancer." *Cancer Treatment and Research* 159: 185–205.

Saad, Bashar, Hassan Azaizeh, and Omar Said. 2005. "Tradition and Perspectives of Arab Herbal Medicine: A Review." *Evidence-Based Complementary and Alternative Medicine* 2 (4): 475–79.

Sam, A. H., V. Salem, and M. A. Ghatei. 2011. "Rimonabant: From RIO to Ban." *Journal of Obesity* 2011: 432607.

Shafi, A., and I. Zahoor. 2021. "Metabolomics of Medicinal and Aromatic Plants: Goldmines of Secondary Metabolites for Herbal Medicine

Research." In *Medicinal and Aromatic Plants*, 261–87. Cambridge, Mass.: Academic Press.

Shao, Q., T. Liu, W. Wang, T. Liu, X. Jin, and Z. Chen. 2022. "Promising Role of Emodin as Therapeutics to Against Viral Infections." *Frontiers in Pharmacology* 13: 902626.

Shipley, Gerhard P., and Kelly Kindscher. 2016. "Evidence for the Paleoethnobotany of the Neanderthal: A Review of the Literature." *Scientifica* 2016: 8927654.

Short, Roger. 2010. "A Plague of People." *Cosmos* magazine, May 13, 2010.

Shoshitaishvili, B. 2021. "From Anthropocene to Noosphere: The Great Acceleration." *Earth's Future* 9 (2): e2020EF001917.

Shuttleworth, A., and S. D. Johnson. 2009. "A Key Role for Floral Scent in a Wasp-Pollination System in *Eucomis* (Hyacinthaceae)." *Annals of Botany* 103 (5): 715–25.

Simard, Suzanne, David A. Perry, Melanie D. Jones, David D. Myrold, Daniel M. Durall, and Randy Molina. 1997. "Net Transfer of Carbon between Ectomycorrhizal Tree Species in the Field." *Nature* 388 (6642): 579–82.

Soulaidopoulos, S., A. Tsiogka, C. Chrysohoou, E. Lazarou, K. Aznaouridis, I. Doundoulakis, D. Tyrovola, et al. 2022. "Overview of Chios Mastic Gum (*Pistacia lentiscus*) Effects on Human Health." *Nutrients* 14 (3): 590.

Stahnisch, Frank W., and Marja Verhoef. 2012. "The Flexner Report of 1910 and Its Impact on Complementary and Alternative Medicine and Psychiatry in North America in the 20th Century." *Evidence-Based Complementary and Alternative Medicine* 2012: 647896.

Stansbury, Jill. 2018-2021. *Herbal Formularies for Health Professionals*. 5 vols. White River Junction. Vt.: Chelsea Green.

Stearn, William T. 1973. *Botanical Latin*. 2nd ed. Exeter, U.K.: David & Charles.

Svarstad, Hanne, Hans Chr. Bugge, and Shivcharn S. Dhillion. 2000. "From Norway to Novartis: Cyclosporin from Tolypocladium Inflatum in an Open Access Bioprospecting Regime." *Biodiversity and Conservation* 9 (11): 1521–41.

Tewari, D., A. M. Stankiewicz, A. Mocan, A. N. Sah, N. T. Tzvetkov, L. Huminiecki, J. O. Horbańczuk, and A. G. Atanasov. 2018. "Ethnopharmacological Approaches for Dementia Therapy and Significance of Natural Products and Herbal Drugs." *Frontiers in Aging Neuroscience* 10: 3.

Tucker, Arthur O., and Sharon S. Tucker. 1988. "Catnip and the Catnip Response." *Economic Botany* 42 (2): 214–31.

Tuli, H. S., M. J. Tuorkey, F. Thakral, K. Sak, M. Kumar, A. K. Sharma, U. Sharma, A. Jain, V. Aggarwal, and A. Bishayee. 2019. "Molecular Mechanisms of Action of Genistein in Cancer: Recent Advances." *Frontiers in Pharmacology* 10: 1336.

UNDRR (United Nations Office for Disaster Risk Reduction). 2022. *Global*

Assessment Report on Disaster Risk Reduction 2022: Our World at Risk: Transforming Governance for a Resilient Future. Geneva: United Nations Office for Disaster Risk Reduction.

Unsicker, Sybille B., Grit Kunert, and Jonathan Gershenzon. 2009. "Protective Perfumes: The Role of Vegetative Volatiles in Plant Defense against Herbivores." *Current Opinion in Plant Biology* 12 (4): 479–85.

Upton, R., ed. 2009. "Skullcap Aerial Parts (*Scutellaria lateriflora*) Monograph and Therapeutic Compendium." In *American Herbal Pharmacopoeia*, 39. Scotts Valley, Calif.: AHP.

USDA (United States Department of Agriculture). 2024. *Longleaf Pine Ecosystem Restoration.* Washington, D.C.: United States Department of Agriculture.

Vauzour, David, Katerina Vafeiadou, Ana Rodriguez-Mateos, Catarina Rendeiro, and Jeremy P. E. Spencer. 2008. "The Neuroprotective Potential of Flavonoids: A Multiplicity of Effects." *Genes & Nutrition* 3 (3): 115–26.

Velasquez-Manoff, M. 2017. "The Self-Medicating Animal." *New York Times Magazine*, May 18, 2017.

Wade, D. T., and P. W. Halligan. 2004. "Do Biomedical Models of Illness Make for Good Healthcare Systems?" *BMJ* 329 (7479): 1398–401.

Wainwright, M. 2002. *The Natural History of Costa Rican Mammals.* Costa Rica: Zona Tropical.

War, A. R., H. C. Sharma, M. G. Paulraj, M. Y. War, and S. Ignacimuthu. 2011. "Herbivore Induced Plant Volatiles: Their Role in Plant Defense for Pest Management." *Plant Signaling and Behavior* 6 (12): 1973–78.

WHO (World Health Organization). 2006. *WHO Monographs on Selected Medicinal Plants.* Vol. 4. Geneva: World Health Organization.

WHO. 2022. *World Malaria Report 2022.* Geneva: World Health Organization.

Wilhelm, R., and C. F. Baynes. 1950. *The I Ching.* Trans. Cary F. Baynes. New York: Pantheon.

Willcox, Merlin, Gerard Bodeker, Phillippe Rasoanaivo, and Jonathan Addae-Kyereme. 2004. *Traditional Medicinal Plants and Malaria.* Boca Raton, Fla.: CRC Press.

Willis, Kathy J. 2017. *State of the World's Plants 2017.* London: Royal Botanic Gardens, Kew.

Wink, Michael. 2008. "Evolutionary Advantage and Molecular Modes of Action of Multi-Component Mixtures Used in Phytomedicine." *Current Drug Metabolism* 9 (10): 996–1009.

———. 2018. "Plant Secondary Metabolites Modulate Insect Behavior-Steps Toward Addiction?" *Frontiers in Physiology* 9: 364.

Wink, Michael, and Oskar Schimmer. 2010. "Molecular Modes of Action of Defensive Secondary Metabolites." In *Annual Plant Reviews*, volume 39:

Functions and Biotechnology of Plant Secondary Metabolites, 21–161. John Wiley & Sons.

Wiser, Mark F. 2022. "Protozoa." In *Reference Module in Life Sciences*. Amsterdam: Elsevier.

Wolfson, P., and D. L. Hoffmann. 2003. "An Investigation into the Efficacy of *Scutellaria lateriflora* in Healthy Volunteers." *Alternative Therapies in Health & Medicine* 9 (2): 74–78.

Wolschke-Bulmahn, J. 1995. "Political Landscapes and Technology: Nazi Germany and the Landscape Design of the Relchsautobahnen (Reich Motor Highways)." In *Selected CELA Annual Conference Papers: Nature and Technology*, Iowa State University, September 9–12, 1995, vol. 7.

Wood, George B., Franklin Bache, H. C. Wood Jr., Joseph P. Remington, and Samuel P. Sadtler. 1883. *The Dispensatory of the United States of America*. 15th ed. Philadelphia: Lippincott.

WWF (World Wildlife Fund). 2021. "One-Third of Freshwater Fish Face Extinction and Other Freshwater Fish Facts." World Wildlife Fund website, February 23, 2021.

WWF (World Wildlife Fund). 2022. *Living Planet Report 2022: Building a Nature-Positive Society*. Edited by R. E. A. Almond, M. Grooten, D. Juffe Bignoli, and T. Petersen. Gland, Switzerland: World Wildlife Fund.

Xiang, L., Z. Chen, S. Wei, and H. Zhou. 2022. "Global Trade Pattern of Traditional Chinese Medicines and China's Trade Position." *Frontiers in Public Health* 10: 865887.

Xiong, Xing-Jiang. 2018. [Treatise on febrile diseases and critical care medicine: exploring connotation of original, dosage, and essence of six meridians from perspective of critical care medicine and integrative medicine]. Article in Chinese. *Zhongguo Zhong yao za zhi* 43 (12): 2413–30.

Yan, Shikai, Run-Hui Liu, Hui-Zi Jin, Xin-Ru Liu, Ji Ye, Lei Shan, and Wei-Dong Zhang. 2015. "'Omics' in Pharmaceutical Research: Overview, Applications, Challenges, and Future Perspectives." *Chinese Journal of Natural Medicines* 13 (1): 3–21.

Yao, R., M. Heinrich, B. Zhang, X. Wei, Y. Qi, and W. Gao. 2023. "Single Botanical Drugs in the Ayurvedic Pharmacopoeia of India: A Quantitative Ethnobotanical Analysis." *Frontiers in Pharmacology* 14: 1136446.

Zhao, Z., P. Guo, and E. Brand. 2012. "The Formation of Daodi Medicinal Materials." *Journal of Ethnopharmacology* 140 (3): 476–81.

Index

About the Author

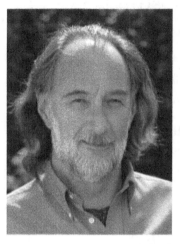

David Hoffmann, FNIMH, RH(AHG), is an internationally renowned medical herbalist. A fellow of Britain's National Institute of Medical Herbalists, he started his herbal practice in Wales in the 1970s, continued at the Findhorn community in Scotland, and has been practicing in California since 1986. A longtime activist in the environmental and peace movements, he ran for parliament in Britain for the Green Party in 1983. He is one of the founding members and a past president of the American Herbalists Guild and has served on the advisory boards of the American Botanical Council, *HerbalGram*, and United Plant Savers.

Hoffmann has taught phytotherapy throughout the English-speaking world, including as a faculty member of the California School of Herbal Studies and as a visiting faculty member at Bastyr University, the California Institute of Integral Studies, the National College of Phytotherapy, and the Rocky Mountain School of Botanical Studies. In 2004 he began working with the wellness company Traditional Medicinals as formulator and principal scientist.

Hoffmann is the author of eighteen books, including the highly regarded *Medical Herbalism*, *The Complete Illustrated Holistic Herbal*, *Herbs for Healthy Aging*, and *The Herbal Handbook*.

Books of Related Interest

The Herbal Handbook
A User's Guide to Medical Herbalism
by David Hoffmann, FNIMH, AHG

An Herbal Guide to Stress Relief
Gentle Remedies and Techniques for Healing
and Calming the Nervous System
by David Hoffmann, FNIMH, AHG

Medical Herbalism
The Science and Practice of Herbal Medicine
by David Hoffmann, FNIMH, AHG

Herbs for Healthy Aging
Natural Prescriptions for Vibrant Health
by David Hoffmann, FNIMH, AHG

The Heart and Its Healing Plants
Traditional Herbal Remedies and Modern Heart Conditions
by Wolf-Dieter Storl, Ph.D.

Adaptogens
Herbs for Strength, Stamina, and Stress Relief
by David Winston, RH(AHG)
with Steven Maimes

Adaptogens in Medical Herbalism
Elite Herbs and Natural Compounds for
Mastering Stress, Aging, and Chronic Disease
by Donald R. Yance, CN, MH, RH(AHG)

Sacred Plant Medicine
The Wisdom in Native American Herbalism
by Stephen Harrod Buhner
Foreword by Brooke Medicine Eagle

INNER TRADITIONS • BEAR & COMPANY
P.O. Box 388
Rochester, VT 05767
1-800-246-8648
www.InnerTraditions.com
Or contact your local bookseller